D0527405

DIET REHAB

28 DAYS

TO BEAT FOOD CRAVINGS AND LOSE WEIGHT

Dr Mike Dow

with Antonia Blyth

MICHAEL JOSEPH
an imprint of
PENGUIN BOOKS

MICHAEL JOSEPH

Published by the Penguin Group
Penguin Books Ltd, 80 Strand, London WC2R 0RL, England
Penguin Group (USA) Inc., 375 Hudson Street, New York, New York 10014, USA
Penguin Group (Canada), 90 Eglinton Avenue East, Suite 700, Toronto, Ontario, Canada M4P 2Y3
(a division of Pearson Penguin Canada Inc.)
Penguin Ireland, 25 St Stephen's Green, Dublin 2, Ireland (a division of Penguin Books Ltd)
Penguin Group (Australia), 250 Camberwell Road, Camberwell, Victoria 3124, Australia
(a division of Pearson Australia Group Pty Ltd)
Penguin Books India Pvt Ltd, 11 Community Centre, Panchsheel Park, New Delhi – 110 017, India
Penguin Group (NZ), 67 Apollo Drive, Rosedale, Auckland 0632, New Zealand
(a division of Pearson New Zealand Ltd)
Penguin Books (South Africa) (Pty) Ltd, 24 Sturdee Avenue,
Rosebank, Johannesburg 2196, South Africa

Penguin Books Ltd, Registered Offices: 80 Strand, London WC2R 0RL, England

www.penguin.com

First published in the United States of America by Avery, an imprint of the
Penguin Group (USA) Inc. 2011
First published in Great Britain by Michael Joseph 2012
2

Copyright © Dr Michael Dow Media Enterprises, Inc., 2011

The moral right of the author has been asserted

Every effort has been made to ensure that the information contained in this book is
complete and accurate. However, the ideas, procedures and suggestions contained in this book
are not intended as a substitute for consulting with your physician.
All matters regarding your health require medical supervision. The publisher is not responsible
for your specific health or allergy needs that may require medical supervision. The publisher
is not responsible for any adverse reactions to the recipes contained in this book.
Neither the authors nor the publisher shall be liable or responsible for any loss or damage
allegedly arising from any information or suggestion in this book

All rights reserved
Without limiting the rights under copyright
reserved above, no part of this publication may be
reproduced, stored in or introduced into a retrieval system,
or transmitted, in any form or by any means (electronic, mechanical,
photocopying, recording or otherwise), without the prior
written permission of both the copyright owner and
the above publisher of this book

Printed in Great Britain by Clays Ltd, St Ives plc

A CIP catalogue record for this book is available from the British Library

ISBN: 978–0–718–15827–9

MIX
Paper from
responsible sources
FSC
www.fsc.org FSC™ C018179

LIBRARIES NI	
C700865078	
RONDO	03/01/2012
613.25	£ 12.99
OMAOMA	

CONTENTS

Introduction. How I Kicked My Food Addiction . . .
and How You Can, Too   1

PART I

Understanding Food Addiction

1. Willpower Is Not the Problem   13

2. How Food Addiction Makes You Fat   28

3. The Secret of Gradual Detox   44

PART II

Your Brain on Food

4. Feeling Anxious: Hungry for Serotonin   71

5. Feeling Blue: Ravenous for Dopamine   101

6. Feeling Powerless: Starving for Everything   127

PART III

Free Yourself from Food Addiction

7. Obsessive Eating: Seeking Security   **141**

8. Emotional Eating: The Search for Joy   **154**

9. Binge Eating: Regaining Control   **166**

PART IV

Rehab Your Diet

10. Change Your Tastes, Change Your Body   **181**

11. Salt Junkies: Hooked on the Gateway Drug   **193**

12. Starved for Serotonin: Jonesing for Sugar and Carbs   **201**

13. Dopamine-Deprived: Longing for Fat and Caffeine   **216**

14. Diet Rehab: The Program   **231**

Appendix A. 7 Days of Quick and Easy Recipes   **297**
Appendix B. Exceptions: Who Should
    Not Use Diet Rehab   **304**
Acknowledgments   **306**
Bibliography   **308**
Index   **315**

DIET REHAB

How I Kicked My Food Addiction . . . and How You Can, Too

'm going to make a confession: I used to have a food addiction. And although I've since kicked the habit, every so often I want one of the foods I used to be addicted to.

Although I eat healthily, work out, meditate, and practice yoga, there are still times when I just feel blue. And sometimes—after I've called a friend, done some deep breathing, or found some other healthy alternative—I still feel desperate for a boost. It's then that I turn to my own secret treat: a big bowl of macaroni and cheese.

Now, I'm not talking about the homemade gourmet "gratin" with four types of *fromage* and a panko crumb crust. I'm talking down and dirty: the 89-cent box you get at the convenience store, the type of gluey treat that you make from elbow macaroni and that grainy orange powder. Sometimes I don't even stir all the lumps out of the sauce. In my late-night slump, those salty little nuggets are actually comforting.

I said I *used* to have a food addiction, and I meant it. I don't turn to my secret indulgence all that often, and because I enjoy it in moderation, it doesn't concern me. My mac and cheese is an occasional treat, not a habitual form of self-medication. But I had wondered many times over the years what it was about that starchy dish that I found so restorative. We all know the term "comfort food," and many of us have felt the pull of a sugar craving, but why? How do these foods affect our feelings? Why would I turn to a carb-laden meal when I needed comfort and calm? And what's the link between emotions, food, and our difficulties with weight?

Then I became a psychotherapist who specializes in disordered eating and addictive behaviors. I began to learn more about how the mind responds to food, which gave me valuable insight into my patients and myself. I discovered that anxiety depletes our store of serotonin, a "feel-good" brain chemical that helps to soothe worries, boost self-confidence, and create a feeling of "okayness" in the world. I also learned that depression and listlessness can signal a shortage of dopamine, the energizing biochemical we all need to function during stressful situations and exciting challenges.

The basics of brain chemistry explained what was happening when I felt anxious or sad. But why did I crave mac and cheese? Why do some people crave high-fat foods while others want starchy carbs or sugary treats in times of stress or sadness?

I began to investigate the way that food and brain chemistry interact, and what I found had that "aha" quality of any discovery that seems to explain a major aspect of your life. I discovered that the carbs in my beloved treat release a quick, feel-good dose of serotonin, and that the high fat content of that neon-orange cheese boosted my dopamine levels. That soothing, calm, and energizing lift wasn't only in my imagination. I really *was* experiencing a chemical reaction, just as if I'd taken drugs to counter my low feelings.

Significantly, both prescription meds and street drugs boost serotonin and dopamine. Prozac and Zoloft, antidepressants that are effective for treating anxiety, increase the amount of serotonin available for our brains to use, while the street drug Ecstasy (MDMA) floods our brain with it, producing that over-the-top, blissed-out, "everything is fabulous" sensation that we've all seen portrayed in movies and on TV. Who knew that pasta, white bread, and doughnuts were cheap, quick, and legal ways to get a mini-version of the same high?

Likewise, the antidepressant Wellbutrin lifts dopamine levels, as do nicotine, amphetamines, and cocaine. But so do bacon, potato crisps, and other high-fat foods.

I realized that when my patients talk about self-medicating with food, it isn't just a metaphor. They really are altering their brain chemistry—often in much-needed ways. It doesn't matter if their low levels of feel-good chemicals were inherited or are the result of a traumatic series of life events. They just know that they don't want to feel as bad as they're feeling.

When people would talk about food addictions, I realized that it wasn't a metaphor. Just as you can become dependent on a nicotine fix or a cocaine high, so can you grow to rely on the effects of high-carb or high-fat foods.

So that was *why* I had turned into a food addict. But *how* had it happened?

How I Became a Carb Junkie

I was fifteen years old when my family changed forever. We were on vacation in Las Vegas. One morning we were walking through the hotel lobby, headed on a daylong trek to a national park, when my ten-year-old brother, David, suddenly vomited. My mom urged me and the rest of my family to go ahead while she stayed behind to nurse my brother through whatever virus he'd picked up. He didn't seem to be in such bad shape, so we thought it was okay to leave.

This was in the days before everyone had a cell phone, and we were gone eight hours. When we returned, they weren't at the hotel. They were in the intensive care unit at a nearby hospital. There I was greeted with a shocking sight: my little brother hooked up to machines and covered in tubes, unable to speak a word. When his eyes found me, he let out an unearthly wail I'll never forget. David had had a massive stroke right after we left.

I stared at him, unable to move. Then I heard a terrible sobbing. It was coming from my strong, unshakable grandfather as he stood beside my brother's bed.

In that moment, everything I thought about adults being infallible simply collapsed. I would never again feel safe as a child. I also knew that I had to be the most perfect, most helpful son in the world. How could my family survive if I wasn't?

Our three-day vacation turned into a three-month stay as we waited for my brother to be released from the hospital. I remember going to some Vegas mall with my mom so she could have something else to wear besides the three changes of clothes she had brought for our brief trip. Suddenly she started crying, unable to figure out what to buy. So there I was, picking out blouses and pants for my mother, terrified to think that *she* was depending on *me*.

My anxiety levels were off the charts and would stay that way for the next several years. Even now this is a part of my psychology and always will be, although I have learned to understand and manage it.

It was eight years and several surgeries before my brother, the victim of a rare brain disease, would improve. He still had only limited use of his right arm. I spent those formative years eating crisps, rice, and pasta. I learned how comforting mac and cheese could be—a whole box could actually calm me down. I lifted my spirits with five or six cans of full-sugar soda a day, and I suppressed my constant worries with a never-ending parade of snacks. My lunch at school every day was a huge bag of fries, and I popped Now and Laters as if they were pills. Sitting alone at the kitchen table while my mom took my brother to endless hospital appointments, I'd find solace in chomping through a massive bowl of ramen noodles.

To make matters worse, our family had been living a dream life in Hawaii until my parents' divorce moved us to Ohio. In Hawaii, we'd gone to nice schools and could have pretty much anything we wanted.

I fit right in, and with my half-Asian heritage I looked like most of the other kids. Then, in Ohio, no one looked like me, and my classmates called me "chink." I didn't have a clue about football or the team sports that were so important there. They didn't care that I surfed in Hawaii. All they knew was that I looked different, couldn't fit into their world, and talked funny.

Then my father had his first heart attack, leading to bypass surgery. He liked greasy foods, too, though I didn't see the connection at the time. Because of the financial burden of his medical bills and the divorce, we were forced into bankruptcy. Now we were penniless. In the grocery store, my mom said we couldn't have our favorite brand-name cereal. She did the best she could, filling us up on bags of pasta covered in cheap, generic-brand sauce.

Each anxiety fed the next, and those carbs came to be a crutch. With my hand in a bag of crisps, I self-medicated my way through my teens. I also channeled my worries into studying. Getting perfect grades and being the perfect son was the only thing I could think of to make things right at home, even though I believed nothing would ever be right again and I was powerless to fix anything.

Throughout all those years, anxiety ruled my life. Then, when I was eighteen, I moved to California to go to college, and a whole new life began. I finally felt as though I fit in. I was making great friends, talking all night with roommates, going out and socializing. In other words, my life was suddenly full of feel-good things other than food. I started to think about my future and about what I wanted and needed. I didn't feel so driven by the desire to be perfect or the constant worry over what other people thought of me. There was a new feeling in my life: that everything was going to be okay.

In a way, I had created my own early version of Diet Rehab: driving out "pitfall feelings" like anxiety and perfectionism with serotonin-boosting activities like socializing and anticipating a happy future; replacing addictive "pitfall sources" of serotonin such as soda, pasta, and crisps with healthy serotonin-boosting foods. Without even realizing it,

I had established Diet Rehab's central principle: When your life is full of serotonin- and dopamine-boosting activities, and when your thoughts trigger big doses of serotonin and dopamine and the self-esteem, optimism, and energy they bring, you will no longer crave the fix of sweets and starches.

Reveling in my new friends and plans, I stopped bingeing on the foods that had once been my lifeline. Sure, I still enjoyed fries and candy, but I wasn't interested in finishing the bag anymore; I stopped after a taste. Not only didn't I need my medication anymore; I hadn't even had to work at letting it go.

Addicted No More

These days I am twenty pounds lighter. I wake up naturally at nine each morning instead of struggling to respond to the alarm. My previously high cholesterol is now in the healthy range, and I gravitate effortlessly to healthy foods. In fact, I crave them.

I've also found a wonderful profession that allows me to help people who struggle with the same issues that I had once dealt with. I understand the addictive power of food because I've lived through it myself. I became a specialist in every kind of addiction: food, alcohol, substance abuse, and addictive behaviors. As a cognitive-behavioral therapist, I've also learned about the kinds of thoughts that set us up for addiction— the negative, unproductive, and misguided ways of viewing the world that send us rushing to *some* form of medication to stop the pain.

One of the things that strikes me most about food addiction is how easily concealed it is—from the outside world, yes, but also from ourselves. I've seen patients who look wonderful on the outside but are actually living a nightmare as they obsessively count calories and worry over every single bite. Some of my skinniest patients are my most addicted. Even the thin models, gorgeous actresses, and seemingly perfect people I have treated suffer from these addictions. Like the rest of us, however, they don't realize that their seemingly uncontrollable cravings are the result of brain chemistry and the biology of addiction. Instead, like the rest of us, they blame themselves for their mysterious "weakness" and hate themselves for being unable to "do better."

My journey culminates with my experience as cohost and psychotherapist on TLC's hit show *Freaky Eaters*, where I have been able to explore food addictions at their most extreme. After years of working with patients and two seasons of *Freaky Eaters*, I've come to see that food addictions are not a problem of willpower or greed. They are a matter of brain chemistry and needing something in your life. The secret to overcoming them is not self-deprivation or self-blame—it's balancing your brain chemistry with foods and activities that boost the feel-good chemicals you need.

The Taste of Freedom

When I finally understood the nature of food addiction, I was ready to create Diet Rehab: a 28-day plan to free you from your food addictions. Diet Rehab is based on the understanding that we become addicted to food because of the chemicals we ingest: serotonin-boosting carbs and dopamine-boosting fats. So the solution is simple: Add healthier "booster" foods—those that promote a sustainable and nonaddictive release of brain chemicals—along with booster activities to increase the chemicals that our brains crave. That way, we naturally lose interest in unhealthy, addictive "pitfall" foods.

In this book I'll work with you to break the hold of food over your body, mind, and spirit. Diet Rehab will teach you to harness the power of your brain chemistry so that you'll no longer feel like a victim of your fluctuating moods and cravings. You'll restore your balance, your energy, and your well-being. You'll start thinking and acting like a person who's always at a healthy weight. And finally, you will become that person.

How do you get to this happy state? By finding healthier, more effective ways to boost your dopamine and serotonin. Instead of relying on addictive fats and sugars, you can take advantage of healthy versions of serotonin's peace, calm, and "okayness" and of dopamine's energy, excitement, and vivacity.

In Diet Rehab, there's no calorie counting and you won't feel deprived. You can continue eating your favorite snacks—not diet versions of them but the actual foods themselves. After twenty-eight days, you'll find that you just don't want them as much, because your brain is getting natural and healthy boosts of the feel-good chemicals you crave instead of relying upon the foods you've become addicted to. You'll be freed of your food addictions because you'll be able to get all the same mood-boosting effects in healthier ways. Instead of continually self-medicating with your mac and cheese, pizza, crisps, or ice cream, you'll be able to see those foods as an occasional welcome treat.

Now here's the *really* good news: Because of Diet Rehab's unique principle of gradual detox, you will be able to make the transition easily and painlessly. That's because we don't take away *anything* until we've added lots of pleasurable and delicious brain-chemistry boosters into your diet and your life. In fact, I'm going to give you easy-to-use tools to help you along the way. My booster food-swap list offers healthier alternatives to common pitfall foods at a glance and my favorite go-to recipes for delicious, boosting dishes that include pizza and mac and cheese! By the time you start to subtract the addictive foods, you'll be totally hooked on the healthy ones.

How to Use This Book

In Part I, I'll show you how high-fat, high-sugar foods affect your brain chemistry, and how you can find alternate ways to create the same comfort, optimism, and excitement. You'll learn to identify "pitfalls"—the foods and thoughts that set up the addictive cycle—and "boosters"—the foods and behaviors that improve your brain chemistry in a healthy way.

In Part II, I'll help you figure out whether you need to replenish serotonin or dopamine, or both. You'll also learn how to identify the pitfalls in your thinking—the negative and addictive patterns of thought that send you into an emotional downward spiral, depleting the brain chemicals that make you feel good and making you desperate for unhealthy foods that can fix your brain chemistry.

In Part III, I'll teach you how to free yourself from your "pitfall" behaviors and habits—the attitudes and thought patterns that set you up for addiction. I'll show you how to break the power of damaging triggers so that you can finally let go of compulsive eating, emotional eating, and bingeing.

In Part IV, we'll rehab your diet. The gradual detox plan I provide will teach you how to fill your plate with healthy booster foods for these crucial chemicals. At the same time, you'll learn how to fill your schedule with "booster activities"—from yoga to paintballing—that will further raise your serotonin and dopamine levels.

Creating Your Ideal Weight— and Your Ideal Life

One thing hosting TLC's *Freaky Eaters* has taught me is that we all struggle with sorrow and anxiety in different ways. For many of us, that struggle is acted out through food. But the good news is that we have the power to transform both our brain chemistry and our habits of thought. Once we understand how our brains and our minds operate, we can harness their tremendous power to attain our ideal weight, stay there permanently, and create our lives as we would have them.

As a cognitive-behavioral therapist, I'm the person who helps you get to the place you know you want to be. If you're like my other patients, you've already been on at least one diet or maybe several. You're probably tired of them not working—and yet you don't want to give up on yourself and your vision of how good you could look and how great you could feel.

I'm here to tell you that you don't have to. With an understanding of your own brain chemistry and the practice of gradual detox, you can fill your life with so much natural peace, joy, and excitement that you'll never have to self-medicate with food again. Food will return to its rightful place in your life—as a source of nourishment and enjoyment— and your focus will shift to creating and enjoying exactly the life you want.

I know you can get there. In fact, I promise you that you can. So let's get started!

With love and kindness,

Dr Mike

Exceptions

There are several conditions that Diet Rehab is not intended to address, and many circumstances in which it should be used only under a physician's or psychotherapist's supervision. Please see Appendix B for more details.

PART I

Understanding Food Addiction

1

Willpower Is Not the Problem

I think you can properly regard food addiction as somewhat similar to drug addiction. If you can help people to at least reduce their craving levels, you'll contribute a lot to solving the obesity epidemic.

—*Tung Fong, director of metabolic diseases research at drugmaker Merck & Co., in the* Chicago Tribune, *2005*

My patient Rosemary sat across from me, gripping the armrests of her chair and speaking quickly and softly, almost in a whisper. It was as though by muffling her words she could keep them from being true. Although Rosemary had been reluctant to talk about her compulsive eating in previous sessions, she had recently seen an episode of *Freaky Eaters* and had been moved by the plight of my patient on that show—a woman who was addicted to sugar. Perhaps seeing that woman confess to frequent bouts of secret eating gave Rosemary the courage to talk about her own.

"I'm just so ashamed," she kept saying as she detailed her struggles to control her weight. "I don't know how I ever let it get this bad." First, she explained, she had been satisfied with an occasional candy bar at work, a sugar rush that helped her get through the most stressful "deadline days" at the online magazine where she reviewed computer software. Then, she'd started having dessert at lunch—a brownie, a piece of cake, a frosted muffin. Somehow her lunchtime treat had expanded into a dinnertime ritual, then a breakfast Danish, then a second candy bar. Now, Rosemary explained, she was essentially eating sugar all day long, a fact that embarrassed her so greatly that she could barely look at me as she spoke.

"So you think this is all your fault," I said carefully when she fell into a long silence, her hands still gripping the armrests.

"Whose fault is it? Nobody put a gun to my head." She forced herself to meet my eyes.

"I'm just weak," she said bitterly, her voice full of defeat. "I'm weak and disgusting, and I deserve to look the way I do."

I often encounter a sense of shame like Rosemary's, whether my patients are struggling with food addictions or substance abuse. In fact, the feelings underneath both conditions are strikingly similar. Most of us like to feel powerful and in control. Acknowledging an addiction makes us feel weak and helpless. It's as though our brain chemistry, and not us, was suddenly in charge of our destiny.

When my patients can accept that *willpower is not the problem*, they often feel liberated and relieved. When Rosemary understood the brain chemistry of food addiction, she began to view herself with more compassion.

"Maybe I'm being too hard on myself," she told me at one session. "I thought I could just stop eating sweets—and then I didn't understand why I *wasn't* stopping. But you're telling me that I was actually developing a physical addiction to sugar. Like an addict, I needed more and more and more—and if I tried to cut back, I felt so awful I could hardly stand it."

She took a deep breath. "So it wasn't just willpower," she said, repeating the words I had once said to her. "I was actually going through withdrawal."

In fact, Rosemary had been going through a rapid, almost violent detox, certain to produce unpleasant and often painful symptoms that were virtually guaranteed to sabotage her efforts. Later in this book, I'll show you how to go through *gradual* detox, so that your Diet Rehab experience is painless and even pleasurable.

First, though, let's find out what Rosemary learned. Let's understand exactly what it means to be addicted to food.

Scientific Proof: Food Addiction Exists!

In March 2010, the Scripps Research Institute released a ground-breaking study. Rats who were fed high-fat, high-sugar diets of bacon, sausage, chocolate, and cheesecake developed full-blown *food addictions*: actual neurochemical dependencies as powerful as those caused by cocaine. Here was the concrete evidence of what I already knew: My favorite mac and cheese was chemically active. It literally affected my brain, just like nicotine, cocaine, or heroin.

In the study, rats were given different kinds of access to high-calorie foods. Some were limited to only an hour of human treats a day, while others were allowed to eat bacon and chocolate virtually around the clock. While the rats with limited access ate moderately and were able to maintain their weight, the rats with more access quickly became obese—and obsessed.

It was astonishing how far those food-addicted rats would go to maintain their habit. When researchers withheld the junk food and tried to put the rats back on a nutritious diet, the obese rats refused to eat, almost to the point of starvation. The rats would even choose to endure painful shocks to get junk food. Their desperation to stuff themselves with sweet and fatty food and their willingness to endure pain in its service was strikingly similar to those of rats in other studies who had become addicted to cocaine or heroin.

Using special electrodes to monitor the rats' responses, researchers discovered that high-sugar, high-fat foods had changed the animals' brain chemistry—again, in virtually identical ways to cocaine or heroin. Both excessive junk food and other types of drugs overload the brain's pleasure centers. Like Rosemary, the rats needed ever-larger quantities of sweet, fatty food to get the same "high."

We tend to think that food's comfort is an emotional issue and blame ourselves for being childlike or weak. But rats don't have psychological issues, and yet they were behaving exactly like food-obsessed humans. Because of the way the food had altered their brain chemistry, these overweight and food-addicted rats *physically* needed more and more junk food to experience pleasure—or just to feel normal. Unlimited access to these foods had turned them into addicts.

Now here's the even scarier part. After cocaine-addicted rats stopped taking the drug, it took only two days for their brain chemistry to return to normal. For the food-addicted rats in the food study, though, their brain chemistry took *two weeks* to return to normal. In other words, food habits affected the brain *more* than drugs in some ways!

The Scripps study shows that we can no longer view unhealthy eating as a matter of willpower. After all, rats don't have emotional issues, childhood histories, or deep-seated associations between food and love. They know only what their brain chemistry tells them. And the obese rats were hearing the message loud and clear: *Go for the bacon and cheesecake*. This new research suggests that drug addiction and food addiction are products of the same neurobiology. That means that sugar and fat can be as addictive as crack. In some ways, maybe even more so.

The Scripps study also showed that these foods don't *have* to take over our lives, *if* we enjoy them in limited amounts. Remember the group of rats that was allowed to eat only bacon- and cheesecake-type foods for one hour each day? Those rats enjoyed their treats, but they did *not* become addicted. Nor did they gain much weight. They had access to seductive "pitfall" foods—but that access was *limited*. As a result, they never became addicted, and their weights remained normal. In fact, their weight was quite similar to a group of rats who were *never* given "pitfall" foods and who were fed only rat chow. But the rats who had access to high-fat, high-sugar foods round-the-clock experienced immediate weight gain. The rats became obese quickly, and their weight spiraled out of control.

Dopamine: The Body's Energizer

Let's take a closer look at what was going on in the addicted rats' brains. All of us—rats and humans alike—respond to the brain chemical dopamine, an energizing, vitalizing substance that our brains produce in response to pleasure and excitement. When you ride a roller-coaster, gamble for high stakes, or go on a thrilling romantic date, your dopamine levels rise. When you feel listless and bored, your dopamine levels have fallen.

Dopamine is responsible for the rush you feel when you first fall in love. It's also one of the brain chemicals that is stimulated by cocaine. That's why people who use the drug feel jazzed-up, wide-awake, and filled with short-lived pleasure. When you think about how good dopamine makes us feel—whether from healthy sources or unhealthy ones—it's hard not to want to be flooded with it all the time.

But here's the problem: The body was not designed for a twenty-four-hour high, whether from romance, cocaine, or anything else. Sooner or later, what goes up must come down. And too great or too intense a thrill inevitably produces a crash.

If you've just gotten back from your first trip to Paris, for example, maybe you feel a little let down your first day back at work. Paperwork seems mundane. Your favorite TV show seems dull. All you want is to get back to the exciting, dopamine-releasing newness that made your heart sing.

Likewise, coming down from a cocaine high is disappointing at best, painful at worst. You feel tired, listless, and burnt out. You usually feel lower than before you did the cocaine in the first place.

So what causes that crash? In most cases, your brain has used up your dopamine stores too quickly. After a few hours of excitement, your brain just can't keep up. Your dopamine stores temporarily run out, and you have even less than you usually do. You feel flat, listless, exhausted, and let down. Time for a rest, so the brain can make more dopamine.

Ideally, we'll get nice, level doses of dopamine that keep us "up" and happy but that aren't so intense and abrupt that they're followed by a crash. That's what happens normally. But what if, like the rats in the study, you are continually pumping up your dopamine levels with regular infusions of "exciting" high-fat foods? Then, like the rats, you may come to depend on those foods—not for excitement but just to feel normal.

Keeping Your Brain in Balance

Our brains are amazing chemical systems. They are designed to keep a nice, steady balance with just the right chemical levels to keep us happy and allow us to function. We have in our brains pretty much all the chemicals we need to recover from pain, rise to a challenge, enjoy a thrill, or just feel good.

When a biochemical reaction modifies your brain chemistry, however, all sorts of problems occur. Suppose you eat a bacon cheeseburger or a nice big bag of crisps. You've just cued your brain to release more dopamine, which is why you get that short-lived rush of pleasure.

Indulging might be fine if you did it only occasionally. But if you overdo the high-fat foods, your brain chemistry begins to change. The neurons that release, receive, and keep dopamine moving through your brain first become overloaded, then damaged. They can't carry dopamine as efficiently as they once did. As a result, you need greater and greater quantities of dopamine to compensate for these overworked neurons.

Meanwhile, by giving yourself a big, extra jolt of those chemicals, you've confused your brain. Soon, instead of producing its own dopamine, slowly and steadily, it "waits" for that big chemical jolt and then produces a flood of dopamine in response. Gradually, your brain begins to depend on that jolt from the outside. Instead of sticking to its own internal, stable rhythm, it responds to those high-fat jolts.

Now that your dopamine neurons are damaged, you need even more dopamine to feel normal than you did before. That outside jolt—the extra fat in your cheeseburger—has to get bigger and bigger and bigger. Where once a single cheeseburger could give you that dopamine rush, now you need two cheeseburgers and a double order of fries.

extra fat ➞ excess dopamine ➞ overworked neurons ➞ need more dopamine to feel normal ➞ eat more fat ➞ flood the brain with extra dopamine ➞ damaged neurons ➞ need more dopamine to feel normal ➞ eat *more* fat ➞ more flooding ➞ more damage ➞ need even *more* dopamine ➞ eat even more *more* fat

Just as the bingeing rats found out, unrestricted access to high-fat foods creates a vicious cycle. The more you eat, the more you want. Your brain chemistry starts to need ever-higher amounts of the outside substance just to function at all.

So what happens when you eat a fat, juicy cheeseburger every day for six months and then suddenly switch to a nice lean chicken breast on a bed of romaine lettuce? Your brain chemistry is seriously disrupted. Since the cheeseburgers had been helping to flood your system with dopamine, your brain now needs more fat than the average, healthy brain just to get a normal dopamine response. So when that low-fat chicken breast *doesn't* generate lots of dopamine, your brain is at a loss. It needs dopamine but it doesn't have any—and the only way it knows how to get more is to be supplied, once again, with fat.

That's where your cravings begin. That chicken breast might have tasted delicious, but if it doesn't give you huge quantities of unhealthy fat, it leaves you feeling listless, let down, and depressed. As we'll see in Chapter 2, you start to have actual withdrawal symptoms, just like a cocaine addict, including sleep disorders, memory problems, difficulty concentrating, and a general feeling of intense discomfort.

Sooner or later, your brain will realize that it has to start making its own dopamine, and slowly production starts again. But remember how long it took the rats in that study to resume eating normally? Two whole weeks. That's how long it takes your brain to kick back into gear.

Serotonin: Feeling Calm, Peaceful, and Positive

The Scripps study wasn't the only one to deal with food addictions in rats. In 2008, another study confirmed that rats can become addicted to sugar. This study showed rats manifesting responses remarkably similar to those of humans: cravings for the sweet stuff, anxiety-based withdrawal, and then a manic, *increased* desire to binge on sugar.

This time, though, the rats were craving not dopamine but serotonin. Serotonin is the feel-good substance that helps us feel calm, at peace, optimistic, and positive about ourselves. People with low serotonin levels feel anxious and pessimistic and suffer from low self-esteem. Low serotonin levels have been implicated in sleep problems and migraines, as well as in depression and mood disorders such as chronic anxiety and obsessive-compulsive disorder. Interestingly, heroin addicts often report powerful sugar cravings as they try to detox from their addictive substance, suggesting a strong connection between sugar and the pleasure centers that heroin stimulates.

Also interesting is the fact that when people diagnosed with depression are given meds to boost their serotonin levels, they not only cheer up but also begin to feel more optimistic about the future and express higher levels of confidence and self-esteem. Just that simple switch in brain chemistry helps them go from "I'll never find a job; who would want to hire me?" to "You know, there was an ad in the paper that looked interesting—I think I'll check it out." Or perhaps "I'm so fat and ugly, no one will want me" turns into "Actually, I'm a terrific person with a lot of great friends, and I feel hopeful that someday I'll meet a great partner, too." Serotonin is integrally bound up in our view of the world, our predictions for the future, and our feelings about ourselves.

Of course, as a therapist I know that psychotherapy can also change your serotonin levels. And later in this book, we'll talk about ways that you can start to change the self-critical, negative thought patterns that might be holding you back into self-loving, positive messages. It's striking that our brain chemistry has so much to do with whether we are able to generate these messages for ourselves or even hear and believe them from others. If your serotonin stores are low, you can hear all the compliments or good advice in the world, and you may very well feel hopeless or anxious anyway. Boosting your serotonin levels is often crucial to any other kind of psychological progress.

So how do you boost your serotonin levels? Sugar will do it—temporarily. So will starchy "sugar-rush" foods made primarily from white or processed flour, including pasta, crackers, breadsticks, and white bread. Of course, foods made with processed flour *and* sugar, such as cookies, cakes, doughnuts, and other baked goods, offer a kind of double-whammy. And, as with the unhealthy dopamine boosters we just looked at, the sugar high is inevitably followed by a sugar crash. After the sugar wears off, you feel *worse* than you did before. You have to keep eating more and more sugar just to get the same high—and eventually, just to feel normal.

Most of us are aware that sweets and starches feel comforting, but we've probably come to believe that's an emotional reaction. Maybe so, but its roots are definitely physical. In a brain-scan study conducted in 2004, scientists found that just the sight and thought of ice cream stimulated the same brain pleasure centers in healthy people as pictures of crack pipes did for drug addicts. Both eating food and thinking about it are deeply biological experiences as well as profoundly emotional ones. If we *feel* addicted to food, it's because we *are*.

Diets Don't Work—Tackling Addiction Does

People aren't stupid. Most of us know that when we feel blue, stressed, or out of control, we eat. That's why we feel so bad about not sticking to a healthy diet. "I *know* this isn't good for me," we tell ourselves. "But I can't control myself! What's *wrong* with me? Why am I so weak?"

Well, now you know that you aren't weak at all—you're simply responding to your own brain chemistry. Overconsumption of high-fat or sweet and starchy foods has taught your body to stop making enough of its own dopamine or serotonin, while tolerance has caused you to need ever-greater quantities of those tempting foods just to feel normal. Take away the addictive foods too suddenly and, like a cocaine addict, you'll go into withdrawal. And your symptoms won't last for just a few days. They'll go on for *two weeks*.

Later in this book, I'll tell you how you can prevent withdrawal symptoms and maintain your brain chemicals so that you never have to feel deprived or uncomfortable while you are changing your diet. But I hope now you're beginning to see why all your other diets haven't worked so well. All those other diets relied on willpower. "If only we can be disciplined," we tell ourselves. "If only we could stop being so lazy and so greedy!" So we South Beach, Atkins, calorie-count, and Blood Type diet our way to insanity. Do you know anyone who has sustained a no-carb diet for years? I don't. Restrictive diets are unrealistic in the long term, and they also make us more likely to gain weight when we do eat. Animal studies have shown that if you radically restrict energy intake—as with a very low-calorie diet—the body's cells go into "starvation mode," trying to conserve all the energy they can.

Then, when you begin eating normally again, your metabolism goes haywire and hangs on to the calories for dear life. Your poor body thinks it's starving and won't give up a single ounce of fat.

So many of us have experienced this effect firsthand. Our bodies learn to conserve weight by going into storage mode. Suddenly we're slipping into a painful downward spiral:

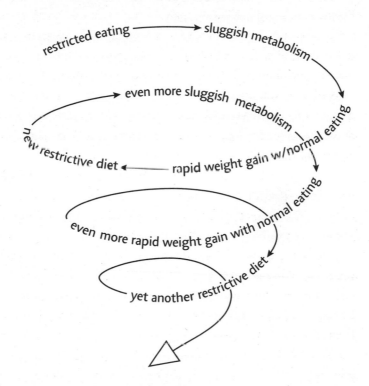

Even after you've had some success on a particular diet—even if that diet offers you healthy choices and a sustainable number of calories—you probably found yourself slipping after a few months. Why?

Again, it's not that you lack willpower. It's that you never focused on feeding your brain. Without the physical and emotional support you need, your brain is starving for the serotonin you got from carbs and sugar and desperate for the dopamine in your fatty snacks.

If your life is stressful or if you feel chronically anxious and unsafe, your serotonin levels probably have been low for a while, making you all the more vulnerable to the power of sugar and carbs. Likewise, if your life feels boring and restricted, if you chronically feel blue and lethargic, your dopamine levels have likely dropped even before you started worrying about your weight.

So what's the solution? It's actually simple. You need healthy, feel-good foods and satisfying life activities to balance your brain chemistry. Once your brain is fed, you won't *need* sweet, starchy, high-fat foods to feel good, because you'll be getting all the "boost" you need from other sources. Your cravings will be satisfied and your addictions will vanish. You'll naturally be drawn to healthy foods, and your weight will automatically readjust.

How Diet Rehab Will Help

As part of your Diet Rehab treatment I'm going to do something that might seem a little strange at first: I'm going to start by having you eat *more* food. My approach to addiction is based on "gradual detox," in which you begin by adding foods that will boost your serotonin and dopamine levels before you ever cut back on *anything*. It's vital that we come from a psychological place of plenty. We need to start out knowing that there is nothing we cannot have if we really want it.

Here's how forcing ourselves to diet cold turkey creates a weight-*gain* cycle:

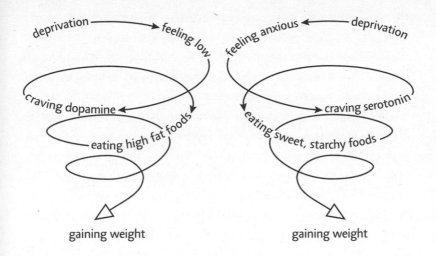

deprivation → feeling low

feeling anxious ← deprivation

craving dopamine ←

craving serotonin →

eating high fat foods

eating sweet, starchy foods

gaining weight

gaining weight

If I'm treating patients who want to quit smoking, I tell them they should continue to smoke for a month after making the decision to quit. I realize that might sound odd, but I'll explain. A habit is fully formed in twenty-eight days. So we spend twenty-eight days *adding* to their life before we take the smoking away. We add activities such as running, yoga, and improving relationships. We start to explore the replacement options we'll have on hand once the smoking stops, such as the medication Zyban, which is yet another way to increase dopamine levels to counteract the effects of nicotine withdrawal. We'll also consider nicotine replacement in the form of gums or patches.

Can you see what we've used that month to do? Nicotine addicts have now formed new habits that boost the same neurochemicals they have gotten from smoking. After raising these levels, then—and only then—should we remove the nicotine from their system. At that point, the smokers will hardly notice the loss, because they'll be getting so much dopamine from so many other sources.

The same principle applies to food. Even when you perform weight loss surgery, if you don't address patients' brain chemistry, they'll continue to feel miserable and deprived. They'll still crave the foods that made them feel good—that did, actually, generate the brain chemicals that we all need to feel good—and then, as happens to most people who have weight loss surgery, they aren't able to stick to the recommended behavioral changes just one year after the procedure. We all have to feed our brains with the right foods and activities or we'll never be able to be free from the addiction.

Diet Rehab *will* address your brain chemistry. You'll learn how to naturally boost your serotonin and dopamine levels, creating the feelings of peace, calm, excitement, and pleasure that you used to get mainly from food. When your brain chemistry is balanced, you'll be interested in food for pleasure, yes, but you won't be dependent on it. It will finally return to its rightful place in your life—and your new weight will show it.

Don't Call Domino's!

The frustrating thing about the food culture we live in is that it's so easy to overexpose ourselves to high-fat or high-sugar/carb foods without even realizing it. For example, in 2010, Domino's made a change that resulted in a huge spike in sales: They changed the recipe of their pizzas to include 40 percent more cheese. Just one slice of the new version contains as much as two-thirds of a day's maximum recommended amount of saturated fat— and how many people stop with just one slice?

Not only does saturated fat put us at risk for heart disease, but, as we just saw, it ramps up our dopamine levels and can trigger an addiction. Might that explain, at least in part, why Domino's sales have risen sharply since the new fattier version hit the menu? Or that pizza is the world's most popular food?

Finding Freedom from Food

I remember the first time I helped free someone from a food addiction. My patient Michelle—a longtime sugar addict—and I had been working for weeks on creating new, healthy habits to drive out the old, addictive behaviors. For a while, as in any process of recovery, it was tough going. Michelle was a fighter—no question about that—but although she was not yet thirty, she had been through a lot: an intense battle with stomach cancer, a subtly abusive boyfriend, and a long string of dead-end jobs.

Now she was finally working in an office where her boss and colleagues appreciated her, and she was looking at programs for going back to school. For the first time in years she wasn't dating, which she viewed as her chance to come into her own and discover who she was. She had recently joined a softball team, started cooking more often, and had just about reached her ideal weight.

One day she burst into my office, grinning from ear to ear. "You'll never guess what happened," she began, before I even had a chance to ask her how she was. "I was walking by my favorite bakery—and I was thinking so hard about this new project at work, and this idea I had for what they could do, and the way I was going to convince them to put me in charge, that I walked right past it! I've never done that before! I didn't even notice. I even told myself that I could go back, if I wanted to, and get myself a doughnut—I've been pretty on target lately, and it was time for a treat—but you know what? I just didn't feel like it. Dr Mike, I can't believe it! I never thought I just wouldn't feel like eating sugar!" Michelle was describing freedom from addiction, and for her it was a beautiful feeling.

Are you wondering whether that could ever be you? Don't worry—I promise you that it can. If you're eager to get started, turn to page 231 and begin your 28-day Diet Rehab. But I'd love for you to read through the next few chapters, because the more fully you understand what is going on in your brain and body, the better choices you'll be able to make and the more motivated you'll be to carry them out.

2

How Food Addiction Makes You Fat

My patient Sondra was a tall, striking woman whose blond hair fell to her shoulders in long, flowing waves. She worked out regularly at her gym, taking a thrice-weekly spin class and lifting weights with a personal trainer. Every morning she carefully prepared a healthy breakfast of egg whites and half a grapefruit, and every afternoon she ate the salad with grilled chicken that she had brought to work from home.

Yet Sondra was at least forty pounds overweight, and she had gained fifteen of those pounds in the past three months.

"I was doing okay there for a while," she told me, trying to smile through what was obviously a difficult conversation. "I was on a new diet—not Atkins, that was last year; and I did South Beach the year before; and the Zone the year before that! But this one was new, and it was working really great! For a while . . . And then . . ." Her voice trailed off.

"What happened?" I finally asked.

She shook her head. "What always happens," she said flatly. "The new diet works great, I lose a bunch of weight, then something messes me up—my boyfriend or my mom or something at work or—I don't even know what. But all of a sudden, I just can't stick to the new diet anymore, no matter how hard I try, and then—bam!—I start eating chocolate and bacon and muffins and cookies. I really love those black-and-white cookies—you know, with the frosting?—and then I gain back all the weight I lost plus another five or ten pounds on top. Then I start a new diet, lose some of the weight, and feel really great—until I screw everything up again."

Sondra was struggling with a very common aspect of food addiction: yo-yo weight gain. Through sheer determination she would force herself to follow a strict diet, suffering through the pain of withdrawal from high-sugar and high-fat foods until her addiction was seemingly broken. She'd go on to eat a healthy diet, lose some weight, and feel terrific.

Then a crisis would hit—nothing major, necessarily, but the normal wear and tear of daily life. Sometimes she'd have a fight with her boyfriend. Other times her mother would make a new demand, or her boss would set a tough deadline, or she'd stress about her growing credit card debt. The anxiety Sondra felt mounted, along with a sense of gloom about why her life wasn't working out the way she'd planned. These difficult feelings soon became overwhelming, and Sondra would inevitably end up self-medicating—with food.

As I shared with you in the introduction, I myself have turned to food for its soothing power. As long as it's only an occasional choice, I think it's perfectly fine to have our favorite food after a tough day or to indulge in high-cal treats. Because Sondra wasn't getting all the nutrients she needed, however, and because she had never changed her addictive attitudes and behaviors, she had remained vulnerable to food addiction. She might escape them when times were good, but she fell prey to them again when times were hard.

Sondra's challenge was all the more difficult because, of course, food is everywhere. Unlike a substance abuser, she couldn't simply avoid the places where she had once gotten high. She was always going to find high-fat, high-sugar food in her break room at work, in the store on her corner, at her family's Sunday dinners, at her boyfriend's apartment. All the places she might have gone to escape the bad influences of a drug habit were places that beckoned and tempted her to indulge her food habit. As I tell my patients, food is the most socially acceptable drug of choice, making it all the harder to overcome a food addiction and keep our relationship to food in-bounds.

Are You Addicted to Food?

How many of us feel that powerful pull of food and think of our lives as one long battle not to give in? That sense of helplessness doesn't come from lack of willpower or emotional hang-ups. It comes from our body's very real, physical need to restore its serotonin and dopamine levels.

Now that you understand how food affects your brain chemistry, it's time to take a look at your own brain. You may not be used to thinking of yourself as a food addict, but if you're struggling with eating habits or weight, and especially if you keep trying to diet, chances are that your brain chemistry is involved.

Check out the questions below and answer them as honestly as you can. There's a wonderful reward in store for you—a gradual detox program that will allow you to make an effortless transition into a calmer, happier, and healthier relationship to food—not to mention a painless way to achieve your ideal weight. The process starts here—so let's get started!

Discover Your Food Habits

- Is there at least one unhealthy food or beverage that you consume every day?

- Do you panic if you think you might not have access to this unhealthy food or beverage everywhere, such as on vacation or at a restaurant?
- Have you ever felt you might need to cut down on this unhealthy food or beverage?
- Has anyone else suggested you change your eating or drinking habits?
- Do you ever feel guilty after eating or drinking?
- Is this unhealthy food or beverage on your mind within an hour of waking up?
- Do you feel powerless when you have a craving?
- Have you tried but failed to cut back on this item in the past?
- Do you turn to this unhealthy food or beverage when you're feeling low or high, or when you're not even hungry or thirsty?
- Have you felt as though your self-esteem and relationships might be better if you didn't have these cravings?
- Do you seem to think about eating or drinking most of the time?
- Is there a difference between your private and public eating?
- Do you tell yourself you could quit consuming this item whenever you want, even though you've never been able to?
- Do you look forward to the time when you can eat or drink this item?
- Are you envious of people who have a casual attitude to food?
- Do you sometimes enter a trancelike state when you are eating?
- Does most of your eating occur late at night?

IF YOU ANSWERED YES TO:

- **One** of these questions: You show signs of a mild food addiction. Although you are basically in control of your food choices and are able to enjoy food's role in your life, you have moments where it feels as though food, not you, is in control.
- **Two** of these questions: You have a moderate food addiction that is probably affecting your life more than you want it to.

Although you are able to enjoy many aspects of your life, food is an ongoing theme that causes you frequent distress.

- **Three or more** of these questions: You may be in the grip of a food addiction that is affecting virtually every aspect of your life. Food is probably playing a much larger role in your life than you are happy with. It's time to deal with the struggle that has been holding you hostage.

Whatever the results of this test, please don't be hard on yourself. Now that you have understood the role that food plays in your life, you're about to get every tool you need to rewrite that role and restore food to its proper place: as a source of nourishment and pleasure. Once you know the right foods and activities to boost your serotonin and dopamine levels, you will restore your brain chemistry, free yourself from your addiction, and go on to a healthy weight and a satisfying life.

If you're ready to get started this instant, turn to page 231. But many of my patients have found it extremely helpful to know a bit more about how addiction works, so that they can really understand what's going on in their bodies, minds, and spirits as they rehab their diets. If you'd like to join them, read on.

The Dangers of Tolerance

One of the key hallmarks of an addiction is *tolerance:* when you keep needing *more* to get the same high. As we build up tolerance to addictive substances, they don't have the power to give us the same kick they once did. Not only do we need more to get the same high; eventually we need them just to feel normal.

You can see this quite clearly with a caffeine addiction. First you drink a cup of coffee and get a pleasant buzz. You feel a bit more alert and awake for a couple of hours.

Then one cup of coffee barely has any effect, so you up your dose to two. Then eventually you need three, and the buzz isn't quite as powerful. Pretty soon you're drinking coffee several times a day, just to stay awake. From a mild and pleasant stimulant, caffeine has become the only thing standing between you and utter exhaustion.

The same thing happens with addictive foods:

- First you just enjoy them.
- Then you need them. You still enjoy them . . . but it hurts not to have them.
- Finally, you need them desperately, just to feel normal. You might not even enjoy them anymore—but you know you feel lousy without them.

Is it possible to have just an occasional addictive food and *not* get hooked? Sure! The Scripps study rats who were fed sweet, high-fat foods for only an hour a day never made the switch to becoming addicted. Their brains continued to work as they always had because their exposure was not great enough to trigger any change. (Likewise, if you limit your intake of caffeine to healthy amounts, you'll probably keep getting a sustainable energy boost when you do drink coffee.)

The rats that had unlimited access to those high-fat foods, however, developed tolerance. The more they ate, the less they felt it. That's why they couldn't stop eating—and why they couldn't stop gaining weight.

Addiction Prescription

Why can't we simply regulate our brain chemistry through medication? Couldn't we take something to prevent outside stimulants from throwing our brains out of balance?

In fact, low doses of dopamine-blocking drugs have been tried on test groups of people to see if they could affect their alcohol consumption. The treatment did reduce drinking by decreasing the enjoyment people found in it, but unfortunately, the dopamine blockers produced Parkinson's-like tremors. (That's probably related to the fact that Parkinson's lowers your dopamine levels about as far as they will go.)

People with substance-abuse problems frequently get substitute drugs. Heroin addicts receive methadone, smokers use Nicorette, and alcoholics and other drug users are prescribed anti-anxiety drugs—all to help wean them off their primary drugs more slowly. The substitutes blunt or prevent withdrawal symptoms, allowing people to clear their systems and rebalance their brain chemistry without suffering.

Well, guess what? In Diet Rehab, we're following the same effective principle! I'm going to have you detox *gradually* from addictive "pitfall foods" as you fill your diet and your life with foods and activities that naturally boost your supply of healthy brain chemicals. That way, you can overcome your addiction painlessly, and transition effortlessly into a healthy new life.

Making It Through Withdrawal

Besides tolerance, the other hallmark of addiction is *withdrawal*—the pain of giving up an addictive substance that the body has come to rely on. My training at the Betty Ford Center and my current work as the clinical director of therapeutic and behavioral services at The Body Well integrative medical center in Los Angeles have given me an intimate acquaintance with withdrawal symptoms. I know very well how painful the recovery process can be.

Here are some of the most common withdrawal symptoms; they plague food, nicotine, alcohol, and drug addicts fairly equally. Have you noticed any of these symptoms whenever you've tried to change *your* diet?

- problems with memory
- impaired concentration
- changes in sleep patterns
- anxiety
- depression
- fatigue
- increased reliance on other addictions
- moodiness
- irritability
- headaches

Sound familiar? No wonder it's so hard to let go of our favorite treats! We're used to thinking of dieting as an emotional issue or a matter of willpower, and those certainly may be elements in our struggles. But at the same time, you're suffering from profound physical symptoms and from the negative emotions inevitably generated by your unbalanced brain chemistry. Why *wouldn't* you self-medicate those symptoms with your favorite treat?

If a steady diet of sugar, starch, and fat could keep you feeling good, it might be worth risking the weight gain, heart disease, diabetes, and cancer that you're putting yourself at risk of, as well as whatever negative feelings you have as the result of your struggles with weight. Unfortunately, because of tolerance and withdrawal, food addiction is not a stable solution to the problem of unbalanced brain chemistry. You're always going to keep wanting more—and you're always risking withdrawal symptoms the moment you cut back. It's hard to revel in the pleasures of food when food feels like your jailer.

How Stress Can Make You Fat

When you feel stressed, your adrenal glands produce a hormone called cortisol. Cortisol is intended for those times when you have to jump into action, as part of the "fight or flight" response. Cortisol raises your blood pressure, so you'll be alert enough to face impending danger. It also instructs your cells to store fat in your midsection, since your body thinks this impending danger means you'll need a storehouse of fat reserves if you're forced to hibernate in a cave for a week with limited food.

Combine the rush of cortisol with the sugary, starchy foods you might crave under stress, and you have a recipe for insulin resistance, a condition in which your body stops efficiently metabolizing your blood sugar. As a result, more of your calories are stored as fat. You'll have trouble losing weight and you're likely to start gaining.

Initially, cortisol and the other elements of your adrenaline rush speed up your metabolism and suppress your appetite, so you're focused on the danger at hand. But then when the rush wears off, you're super-hungry. That's because your body expected you to burn off all that extra blood sugar and fat running from a charging mammoth or fighting off an invader, so it creates some hunger to compensate for this supposed activity.

But if your emergency was a pressing deadline, a fight with a friend, or a crying baby, your efforts have likely been emotional, not physical. And further, if you've created additional stress through "pitfall" thoughts or attitudes (see page 53), your stress—and your subsequent hunger—will increase. Now you're eating food that your body doesn't really need—although your biochemical reaction is insisting that you're hungry.

Cortisol also suppresses your immune system and depletes your serotonin and dopamine levels, sending you into a state of anxiety and, eventually, nudging you toward depression. Again, cortisol creates biochemical conditions in which you're more likely to turn to food.

Finally, the fat cells around your belly are particularly sensitive to cortisol and to high insulin levels. This area of the body is also very effective at storing energy. That's why excess stress often leads to weight gain on our bellies.

A fascinating study conducted at Yale University found that women with belly fat felt more overwhelmed by stressful tasks and produced more cortisol than women whose fat was stored primarily around their hips. So if you'd like a flatter belly, think about reducing the stress in your life. I'm the first one to agree that that isn't easy—if just saying "reduce stress" were enough, none of us would be stressed! However, I can offer you something more helpful than empty advice: The activities suggested throughout this book to boost your brain chemistry are just the anti-stress tools you need! Boosting your serotonin levels will make you feel calmer and less stressed while giving you more emotional resources to cope with the stress you can't avoid.

Addiction and Yo-Yo Dieting

Suppose, like my patient Sondra, we do make it through two weeks of chemical detox from our high-fat, high-sugar diets, however painful or unpleasant that might be? Suppose, like Sondra, that we've done that not only once but twice, three times, maybe up to a dozen times as we went from diet to diet to diet? Each time we lasted one month, maybe two, maybe even six, making it well past the withdrawal symptoms and maybe even dropping a few pounds. But sooner or later we find ourselves turning to high-fat or sweet and starchy foods, and our diets fail.

Once again, brain chemistry is the culprit. We need to maintain healthy serotonin and dopamine levels to feel good, and if we aren't eating the right foods or engaging in the right activities, our levels will fall too low. We may force ourselves to forgo our "medication" for a few weeks or even a few months. But unless we genuinely learn to replace it with something healthier, we'll always be tempted to come back.

Are You "Naturally" Fat? The Truth About Genetics

Can you be "naturally" fat? The answer is both "yes" and "no."

Yes, up to one-third of the factors that determine body weight can be attributed to our family inheritance. Studies of twins and adopted children have revealed that biological relatives tend to be a similar body weight, even if they grew up in completely different households. First-degree relatives of moderately obese people (fifty to sixty pounds overweight) are three to four times more likely to become obese than people from a different type of family. First-degree relatives of severely obese people (ninety to one hundred or more pounds overweight) are five times more likely to develop obesity. At least some of this correlation seems to be genetic rather than having to do with family eating habits and emotional patterns.

But no, regardless of what anyone else in your family looks like, you don't *have* to be obese—and you don't have to starve yourself to stay thin, either. What you eat, how you exercise, and how you nourish your brain chemistry through both food and activities all play an enormous role in determining your metabolism and your weight.

In 2010, genetic researchers in the United Kingdom studied more than 20,000 people aged between thirty-nine and seventy-nine years. Their conclusion: Thirty minutes of moderate exercise per day can reduce any genetic tendency toward obesity by 40 percent. Other studies have come to similar conclusions.

So here's the bottom line: Regardless of who's in your family, if you undergo Diet Rehab and learn how to feed your brain chemistry, you're well on your way toward achieving your healthy weight, especially if you build in thirty minutes of moderate exercise a day. And guess what? The right kinds of moderate exercise will also feed your brain chemistry, boosting your levels of both serotonin and dopamine. Now that's what I call a win-win!

Getting to Know Your Hunger

I hope you can see by now that if you're at an unhealthy weight, you're responding to brain cues that have nothing to do with your body's need for nourishment.

One of the best ways to address body, brain, and emotion together is to get in touch with your hunger, which is one of the first things I ask my patients to do. I'm going to ask the same of you. As you begin to move through the process of Diet Rehab, I'd like you to ask yourself the following questions each time you feel hungry. Don't judge or blame; just notice.

WHEN DO I FEEL HUNGRY?
—after something upsetting happened
—after something wonderful happened
—because I'm bored
—to take a break
—when I feel like I deserve a reward
—based on a cue: after a TV show is over, when I get home, etc.

HOW DO I FEEL HUNGRY?
—suddenly I'm ravenous
—gradually, my hunger goes from being a small feeling to a progressively greater one
—I crave particular foods or types of food
—I feel desperate
—I feel calm and pleasant anticipation
—I am constantly hungry
—I am constantly looking forward to my next meal
—I look forward to the food itself
—I look forward to some other aspect of the meal: the break, the time with family or friends, the chance to get away from work or out of the house

None of these responses is wrong or bad, though some of them might be signs that your body, brain, or spirit isn't getting something that it needs. Feeling constantly hungry, for example, probably means that you're not nourishing yourself properly, whether you're overly restricting your diet, eating too much sugar or starch (creating blood sugar spikes of "fullness" followed by crashes of feeling ravenous), or otherwise not correctly feeding your brain chemistry. It could also mean that there is a huge emotional hunger in your life that isn't being met—but, as we've seen, that is a brain chemistry issue as well as a physical one.

If we're eating healthy meals and snacks filled with booster foods, usually we'll feel gradual hunger every two to three hours. If we've stuffed ourselves with a big meal, we may not feel physically hungry for at least six hours, as physical hunger usually comes on slowly and gradually. However, as we've seen, if you've been under stress and your cortisol levels have risen, you are likely not to feel hungry as you cope with the problem that stresses you. Then, when the stress is over—when the deadline is met or the baby finally stops crying—you may feel ravenous. That is also a physical response, triggered by your body's response to a stress hormone, but it doesn't necessarily indicate that you need food.

Eating when you're bored, to give yourself a break, on a set schedule, or in response to a cue might mean that you're eating food you don't really need. One study compared Americans to French eaters, showing that the French are more inner-directed when it comes to hunger, listening to their bodies rather than to social cues. Americans, by contrast, ate according to external cues. For example, we tend to stop eating when the TV show we're watching is over or when others have stopped eating.

As you can see, sorting out how, when, and why you feel hungry and how you might best respond is a complicated business, and there are no simple rules or easy answers. However, what will help break the hold of your food addiction is just to notice when, how, and why you feel hungry. Notice your body, your emotions, your schedule, and the cues you might be responding to. Don't judge, blame, or expect yourself to do something; just *notice*.

We'll come back to this question of hunger and your body's cues as we move through the four weeks of Diet Rehab. Later in the program, when you've added serotonin-boosting and dopamine-boosting foods and activities to your diet and your life, you may notice places you'd like to make a change. You might even notice that, naturally and gradually, a change has already taken place.

Gastric Bypass and Lap-Bands: Are They the Answer?

Lap-Bands and gastric bypass surgeries work by physically altering the stomach's capacity. You become unable to eat more than a tiny amount at any sitting—perhaps as little as a small carton of yogurt. If the only problem with out-of-control eating were your capacity to fill your stomach, a gastric bypass or Lap-Band would work well.

The problem is that just restricting your access to food doesn't change the reasons that you were eating excessively in the first place. If your brain chemistry remains unbalanced—if your brain is still jonesing for dopamine and serotonin—keeping yourself from eating too much at one time will not change the dynamic.

Certainly, these surgeries help save lives. Many morbidly obese people have benefited from them. But in my professional opinion, surgery alone is not enough. If you're considering this procedure, it's vital for you to receive psychotherapy for at least six months to help you deal with your emotional connection to food.

In fact, most patients are noncompliant with at least one of the behavioral changes recommended within one year of having bariatric surgery. Many do not adhere to the recommended changes in either diet or exercise. I have treated a number of patients who have had these surgeries and have regained all the weight they initially lost. When this is true, they are putting themselves at risk for complications and can stretch their surgically modified stomachs.

If you're considering either of these procedures, start your psychological preparation before you go. Attend some free 12-step Overeaters Anonymous meetings, commit to a weight-loss group for a year, or go see a therapist for at least six months to figure out whether you can avoid surgery or, failing that, how to prepare yourself emotionally. Don't fall into polarized thinking, where you see only a single "either/or" choice. My own recommendation is to keep the surgery option open while committing to a year of Overeaters Anonymous and individual psychotherapy—that would really be setting yourself up for success.

Bear in mind that after surgery, you're going to be getting less serotonin and dopamine from food than you did previously. That makes it all the more important to follow the diet and lifestyle suggestions in this book, and that you make sure to get more of your feel-good chemicals from booster activities so that you are relying not only on food to keep your brain chemistry balanced.

The Reward Response

There is one other aspect of addiction I'd like you to know about. We've seen that sugar and starchy foods relate to our hunger for serotonin and that high-fat foods feed our need for dopamine. But whenever anything pleasurable happens to us—from receiving a compliment to eating a healthy meal to enjoying a decadent dessert—we also get a little shot of dopamine, a tiny burst of *Yes! That feels good!*

That little bit of dopamine serves as a reward for anything we do that feels good. As you can see from the examples I've chosen, it can be a reward for good behavior or bad, for a healthy choice or an unhealthy one. It's simply our body's way of acknowledging that something felt good—whether that good feeling is "good for us" in the long run or not.

Many of us have struggled with relationships that we know aren't always good for us but that sometimes *feel* good at the time, even if we know there's going to be a price to pay later. When that unavailable or unreliable hottie smiles at you or asks you out, it might feel so good that you're willing to ignore your awareness that he might not show up or that she might let you down later on. That little shot of dopamine often feels so good that it's hard to imagine feeling low later.

Likewise, when a sweet or fatty treat beckons and we take that first bite—or sometimes just *imagine* taking that first bite—we get that little dopamine rush, and it feels wonderful. We can try to picture what comes later, when we feel bloated, frustrated, or annoyed with ourselves, but our present reality is that brain chemical, which gives us an immediate, powerful reward.

This dopamine reward is one of the reasons addictions are so hard to give up, even when we've physically detoxed from them. As we saw earlier, just looking at or imagining a sweet treat can set up powerful responses in our brain, with dopamine kicking in at the very thought of the pleasure we can expect. Even when the physical addiction is broken—when there are no more withdrawal symptoms and our body is back to normal—that dopamine reward beckons, and it can be very hard to resist.

What's the solution? Giving yourself so many other rewarding, nourishing activities and so many healthy dopamine boosters in your diet that those unhealthy choices are no longer your only or your primary source of dopamine-fueled pleasure. When your body and your brain really feel as though you're living in a world of plenty, your addictive responses simply become less interesting, and maybe, eventually, not interesting at all. The solution is not to fight them and blame yourself for having them, but to notice them and learn about them while adding all sorts of other pleasurable choices into your life. That's what Diet Rehab is all about—and that's why it works.

3

The Secret
of Gradual Detox

When Marisa strode into my office, I felt I was in the presence of a force of nature. Short, dark-haired, and intense, she rattled off a series of rapid-fire sentences in a firm, no-nonsense tone. You could tell that this cofounder of a rising new financial services company was used to making things happen—and fast.

Marisa nodded intently as I explained to her the nature of food addictions and the relationship between her brain chemistry and her struggles with weight. But when I shared with her my approach to gradual detox, she balked.

"What do you mean I'm going to spend two weeks adding healthy new foods into my diet before I even begin to cut out the bad foods?" she sputtered. "I don't have time to screw around, Dr Mike. I'm a very disciplined person. Just tell me what to do, and I'll do it."

I could see that Marisa's drive and determination—enormous assets in her business life—were actually getting in the way of her personal development. She had already told me that she'd tried three previous weight-loss plans, each of which had failed. I had the feeling that with all three of them, she'd flung herself into a wildly disciplined regime with a kind of cold turkey approach to food detox. Then, when crises hit, she didn't have the resources to handle them. Her superior discipline crumbled, she returned to all her favorite comfort foods—and then, when her schedule eased up, she looked for another diet.

I didn't want to be one more failure on her list. More important, I wanted to give *her* the chance to create a lasting transformation.

"Marisa," I said, trying to find the words that would get through to her, "you told me that last year you quit smoking. Did you do it cold turkey?"

She looked at me in astonishment. "Of course not. I'm not an idiot! I took Zyban. Even then it was tough—but I did it. I do everything I set my mind to."

"That's terrific," I told her. "And I'm glad you gave yourself so much support while you were trying to give up nicotine. That's exactly what I'm trying to do with your addiction to food. We need to give you lots of support, build up your healthy habits, and ease the pain of withdrawal. That's what gradual detox is all about."

Marisa stared at me in astonishment, then made one of her characteristic quick decisions. "Fine," she said, opening her arms wide in a gesture of surrender. "Let's get started."

What Is Gradual Detox?

As I explained to Marisa, gradual detox is a way of slowly letting go of an unhealthy habit by gradually replacing it with something else, allowing you to circumvent the possibility of withdrawal. One obvious example of gradual detox is when smokers use nicotine gums or patches, or when they take Zyban or other medications. These approaches blunt the agonies of withdrawal either by tapering off nicotine intake slowly or by helping to restart the production of dopamine and other brain chemicals that cigarette smoking has undermined.

Likewise, with Diet Rehab, I'll keep you from feeling any withdrawal symptoms by having you continue to eat the foods you crave. As we've seen in previous chapters, addictive foods inhibit your body's ability to manufacture its own stores of serotonin and dopamine. As a result, when you stop eating them, you feel uncomfortable withdrawal symptoms and crave the addictive foods even more.

With gradual detox, you won't have to subject yourself to that painful period of withdrawal. That's because you'll be adding new foods, activities, and thought patterns to your daily routine, so that you'll have restored your body's ability to manufacture its vital brain chemicals. That way, when you begin to cut back on the addictive foods, your body will be getting all the serotonin and dopamine that it needs. Gradual detox makes the transition from addiction to freedom feel easy and even pleasant.

Did you know it takes at least ten exposures to a new healthy food to accept and then to crave it? That's why Diet Rehab has you adding so many healthy foods to your diet over the twenty-eight days of the program. You're giving your body time to gradually detox from pepperoni pizza and start to crave salmon, to gradually detox from cookies and doughnuts and start to crave blueberries and mangos. Replacing the old unhealthy cravings with healthy new ones will happen gradually and naturally, so that you never experience withdrawal and you never feel deprived.

Gradual detox is based on the understanding that it takes a month for the human brain to create a habit. So during the twenty-eight days of Diet Rehab, you'll be creating healthy new habits—habits that you'll start to cultivate long before you have to give up any of your unhealthy old habits! The five-minute walk in the middle of your work day or the lunch break at that healthy café will become habitual parts of your everyday life.

Pitfalls and Boosters

Gradual detox is accomplished through the two cornerstones of Diet Rehab: *pitfalls* and *boosters*.

Pitfalls are the foods, activities, and thought patterns that ultimately lower your supplies of the brain chemicals you need to feel healthy, happy, and energized. A pitfall food—something high in starch, sugar, or fat—temporarily lifts your serotonin or dopamine levels, but the high is soon followed by a crash, and, as we've seen, these foods undermine your body's ability to make its own stores of these vital brain chemicals.

A pitfall activity is any type of behavior that likewise lowers your stores of vital brain chemicals. As we saw in the previous chapter, high-stress situations can boost your levels of the stress hormone cortisol, which contributes to lowered serotonin and dopamine. A long, boring meeting at work, an unpleasant lunch with a highly critical family member, or an ongoing relationship with someone who doesn't treat you well might all be pitfall activities, lowering your stores of serotonin, dopamine, or both. While you might not always be able to avoid pitfall activities, you can at least be aware that they call for extra brain chemistry support to undo their damage.

We'll look at pitfall thought patterns later in this chapter. These are often hard to recognize as pitfalls, especially if we're used to having them. But if you can let go of your mental pitfalls, you might be amazed at how much better you feel—and at how much better your life becomes.

Boosters are the opposite of pitfalls—they're foods, activities, and thought patterns that boost your stores of serotonin and dopamine, giving you the physical and emotional nourishment that your body, mind, and spirit crave. If one day's diet includes Greek yogurt, berries, brown rice, salmon, and fresh vegetables, you have spent that day boosting your serotonin and dopamine, helping yourself feel calm, optimistic, and energized.

Activities can also boost your brain chemistry. Whenever you take a brisk walk, spend five minutes meditating, chat with a friend on the phone, or learn something new and interesting, you are likewise altering your brain chemistry, boosting your serotonin and dopamine levels, and transforming the way you feel.

Thought patterns can further boost your serotonin and dopamine stores, setting you up for optimism, self-confidence, and joy. Later in this chapter, I'll help you identify some booster thought patterns that you can use to replace your pitfall patterns.

The secret of Diet Rehab can be summed up in two sentences:

1. First add booster foods and booster activities to your life.
2. Then gradually reduce pitfall foods and pitfall thoughts.

That's it. It's that simple. Fill your life with foods, activities, and thought patterns that boost your brain chemistry, and you'll find it remarkably easy to let go of the pitfall foods and thought patterns that have been setting you up for food addictions and weight gain. Once your life is full of boosters, you'll have a much easier time eliminating the pitfalls—and your body will effortlessly adjust to a healthy weight.

Why Diet Rehab Works Where Diets Fail

If you're like most people, pitfall foods are a part of your everyday life, keeping you addicted and coming back for more. I'm sure by the time you've picked up this book, you've tried not once but many times to limit your calories or portions—but to no avail. If you're like the vast majority of people, you've been on diet after diet, all of which have failed in the long run.

Why don't diets work? Because, as we've seen in Chapters 1 and 2, they didn't free you from your addiction to pitfall foods. You'll notice that we don't keep a strict tally of your daily intake of calories or carbs here. Why? Because that's an approach from the outside in that it imposes an external limit upon you. To make matters worse, it doesn't address the withdrawal that you're likely to feel if you try to cut back on pitfall foods abruptly, without addressing your brain chemistry.

To make matters still worse, the outside-in approach is doomed to fail in the long run because, without addressing your brain chemistry, you're going to long for pitfall foods and their temporary but potent effect on your serotonin and dopamine levels. You may be able to resist those longings when things are going well, but when stress or major challenges inevitably reenter your life, you're likely to turn to the old reliable pitfalls that pull you deeper into addiction. What's the result? You feel hopeless, decide you're a failure, and berate yourself for your lack of willpower. This pitfall thinking keeps you trapped in the downward spiral of weight gain and food addiction.

Diet Rehab, by contrast, works from the inside out. I want you to let go of pitfall foods *only when you feel ready to do so*. That's why I haven't even suggested cutting anything back during the first fourteen days of the program. I'll go further—I don't *want* you to cut back. Just add in booster foods and activities. The letting go of your old ways of eating, thinking, and feeling will practically happen by itself.

Adding food to your diet will tackle the root of food addiction through boosters that will help you balance your brain chemistry. The boosters will also help you to improve your life. You'll have both the body you want *and* the life you want, because your healthy, nourished brain will have all the support it needs.

When you've completed Diet Rehab, you'll notice that your addictive cravings will have subsided. Suddenly, adhering to any dietary or caloric restrictions will be doable, because you've worked from the inside out. Since you're now feeding your brain chemistry, you will find yourself wanting to eat less in general. Your body has recalibrated to normal levels. Nothing will be off limits forever, because, as the Scripps study showed, occasional exposure to pitfall foods doesn't cause addiction. Not to mention that saying *"I'll never eat this"* sometimes can make you want it more!

Diet Rehab: 28 Days of Gradual Detox

How does this work in practice? Let's take a look. Here's the basic outline of twenty-eight days of Diet Rehab:

WEEK 1

- **Don't cut anything from your normal diet.** We add before we take away.
- **Make sure that at least *one* of your meals or snacks each day is made up of serotonin or dopamine booster foods.** In Part II you'll determine whether you are serotonin deficient, dopamine deficient, or both. If you need to replenish both types of brain chemical, alternate by adding a serotonin booster meal or snack one day and a dopamine booster meal or snack the next.
- **Add *one* booster activity each day.** Based on your findings in Part II, I'll give you a list of activities that will replenish the neurochemicals you need most. If you need to replenish both serotonin and dopamine, alternate by adding a serotonin booster one day and a dopamine booster the next.

WEEK 2

- **Don't cut anything from your normal diet.**
- **Make sure that at least *two* of your meals or snacks each day are made up of serotonin or dopamine booster foods.** If you need to replenish both types of brain chemicals, add one serotonin and one dopamine booster meal or snack each day.
- **Add *two* serotonin or dopamine booster activities each day.** As with your food boosters, if you're both serotonin and dopamine deficient, add one booster activity for each neurochemical every day.

WEEK 3

• **Limit your pitfall foods to no more than *three* servings per day. The rest of all meals and snacks will be made up of booster foods.** Favor boosters tailored to your brain chemistry, but now that your brain chemistry is beginning to be balanced, any booster food will start to be beneficial. A pitfall food serving should be around 300 calories at most, so you're going for a maximum of about 900 calories from pitfall foods a day.

• **Add *three* serotonin or dopamine booster activities each day.** If you need to replenish both types of brain chemical, alternate between adding two serotonin boosters and one dopamine booster, and adding one serotonin booster and two dopamine boosters.

WEEK 4

• **Limit your pitfall foods to no more than *two* servings per day. Everything else you eat should be boosters.** Favor boosters tailored to your brain chemistry, but now that your brain chemistry is beginning to be balanced, any booster food will start to be beneficial. Remember, one serving of a pitfall is about 300 calories, so you're looking at a maximum of about 600 calories of pitfalls.

• **Add *four* serotonin or dopamine booster activities each day.** If you need to replenish both types of brain chemical, add two boosters of each type every day.

MAINTENANCE

• **Limit your pitfall foods to no more than *two* servings per day. The rest of all meals and snacks will be made up of boosters.** Favor boosters tailored to your brain chemistry, but now that your brain chemistry is beginning to be balanced, any booster food will start to be beneficial. Remember, one serving of a pitfall is about 300 calories, so you're looking at a maximum of about 600 calories of pitfalls.

• **Maintain *four* booster activities each day.** Favor booster activities tailored to your brain chemistry (low serotonin or low dopamine), but now that your brain chemistry is beginning to be balanced, any booster activity will start to be beneficial. Low serotonin types may want to add a few dopamine booster activities, especially when they feel like they need an energizing lift. Low dopamine types may want to add a few serotonin booster activities, especially when they need some peace and calm. Dual-deficiency types can continue to add from both dopamine booster and serotonin booster activities lists.

Looking for a Shortcut?

I'd like you to read every word of this book because I think the more you understand about food addiction and brain chemistry, the more empowered and proactive you'll be at implementing Diet Rehab and making it work for you.

But if you're eager to get started and just want to know exactly what to do, here's how you can move through this book more quickly:

1. Take the quizzes on pages 73 and 105. They will help you figure out whether you are serotonin deficient, dopamine deficient, or both.

2. Based on what you learn about your body chemistry, go to the lists of booster foods and activities on pages 204 and 219. Choose as many as you can and prepare to add them to your daily diet and lifestyle.

3. Go to the list of pitfall foods on pages 213 and 228. Identify which are part of your current regime.

4. Look at the outline on page 50. Select the correct number of booster foods and activities to add and pitfall foods to subtract over the twenty-eight days.

Those are the basics. Add booster foods and activities, gradually increasing them over the twenty-eight days, and, two weeks into the program, start cutting back on your pitfalls until you're down to only two or fewer per day (one pitfall serving is about 300 calories, so you're down to a maximum of 600 calories in pitfalls). If you'd like some additional support in avoiding pitfall types of thinking and adding booster thought patterns, continue reading this chapter.

Pitfall Thought Patterns: The 7 Ps to Avoid

As a cognitive-behavioral therapist, I specialize in identifying thought patterns. You could boil my whole profession down to one simple sentence: Thinking in certain types of patterns makes us feel better, while thinking in other types of patterns makes us feel worse. As a therapist, I help my patients identify the thought patterns that get them into trouble and encourage them to reframe their thoughts into a more helpful approach.

Cognitive-behavioral therapy is actually an integral part of Diet Rehab, because pitfall thoughts hurt your brain chemistry and are also more likely to be a result of low levels of serotonin and dopamine—another example of a downward spiral.

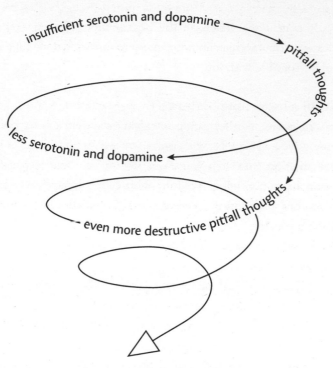

even less serotonin and dopamine

How do pitfall thoughts erode your stores of serotonin and dopamine? By feeding your anxiety, self-doubt, hopelessness, and despair, which lead to behaviors that cause more of these unpleasant feelings. Pitfall thoughts can make you feel helpless, worthless, and unsafe, and they can contribute to feeling stuck, trapped, and bored. As we have seen, these are the feelings that accompany insufficient stores of serotonin and dopamine, which is precisely the brain-chemistry condition that sends you running for cheeseburgers and cheesecake to boost your mood. In fact, even if your diet is filled with terrific booster foods, pitfall thoughts can undo your good habits and push you toward your fat or sugar fix.

Luckily, there is a way to reframe pitfall thoughts, so let me show you how it's done. Then, in the next section, I'll help you identify booster attributes that can raise your serotonin and dopamine levels—and fill your life with joy.

Pitfall #1: Personalization

Personalization is when you assume that something is happening because of you. Of course, sometimes you *are* responsible for a problem or a situation, and then you should realize that and own it. But the personalization pitfall comes into play when you have no explanation or another explanation—yet you still choose the one that involves blaming yourself.

PITFALL THOUGHTS:

"They didn't call me for an interview. I'm not smart enough."

"He didn't call me because I'm too fat."

"This diet isn't working because I have no self-control."

REFRAMED THOUGHTS:

"I really would have liked that job, so I'll keep looking. Perhaps they had already hired someone else."

"I don't know why he didn't call me—maybe he's busy, insecure, or interested in someone else he met before me."

"This diet isn't working—maybe it's time I did things differently and looked at what I need to change."

Here's how you can tell if you personalize something: Just about every explanation for anything that goes wrong begins and ends with you not being good enough.

This kind of thinking can get you into trouble, because in pretty much any circumstance, you're usually only *one* part of the equation, and your failures and shortcomings are only *one* part of you. Personalization blocks out all the aspects of life and relationships that are about other people or circumstances in general. Blaming yourself and taking things personally makes you feel hopeless, helpless, and unworthy.

Now, please don't start blaming yourself for taking things personally! Just try to reframe your thoughts to imagine other explanations. If you really want to avoid this pitfall thought pattern, try one week or even one day when you don't allow yourself to think of "not being good enough" as the reason for *anything*. You might be surprised at all the alternate explanations you come up with!

Pitfall #2: Pervasiveness

Pervasiveness is when any problem in any area of your life invades all the others. If one part of your life goes bad, you shut down in all areas. Of course, this makes *everything* worse because you allowed one weakness to nullify all of your strengths.

PITFALL THOUGHTS:

"I gained some weight this week—I'm calling in sick to work tomorrow."

"He didn't call me—I'm not going to make an effort with him—or my friends, either."

"I'm worried about money—I'm just going to pick up a pint of ice cream."

REFRAMED THOUGHTS:

"I gained some weight this week—but if I go into work tomorrow, I can have lunch with Maria, and she always cheers me up. I also know that once I'm there, I'll probably end up forgetting about most of my frustration."

"He didn't call me—and it's times like these when my friendships are actually more important. Even though I don't really feel like it, I'm going to call a few friends and see if I can schedule some get-togethers."

"I'm worried about money—but the last thing I want to do is be worried about money *and* my health. I'm going to take a ten-minute walk and then focus on what financial changes I can make."

When something goes wrong in one part of our lives, it's easy to let that affect *all* of our life. The antidote to pervasiveness is *perspective*. In the grand scheme of things, your sorrow, frustration, or failure, however painful or upsetting, is only one piece of your life. Don't let it spoil all the rest.

Some people believe that the antidote for pervasiveness is *gratitude*. They go by the maxim, "I was upset that I had no shoes—until I met the man who had no feet." The point of remembering what you have to be grateful for is *not* to undermine your feelings or to mock you for having a hard time. It's to help you remember that there is always something more than the present moment, and always something greater than a single setback or even a whole period of setbacks. Reframing your pervasiveness into a larger vision of your life can help you boost your brain chemistry and regain your balance.

Pitfall #3: Paralysis-Analysis

This pitfall involves getting stuck in your own thoughts, trying to analyze what's wrong with you every time a sad, angry, or unpleasant feeling surfaces. Of course, sometimes it's appropriate to try to figure out a problem or solve a difficult situation. But if you've thought about that problem all you can and either there isn't any solution or there isn't one that you can implement right away, sometimes it's simply better to distract yourself than to ruminate.

PITFALL THOUGHTS:

"What does it mean about me that I can't lose weight?"

"I wonder if my coworker is angry at me. I wonder why it took her so long to answer that e-mail today—what does that mean?"

"I'm feeling blue, and I'm going to sit here thinking about why until I feel better."

REFRAMED THOUGHTS:

"I've done all I can today to work on my weight-loss issues—now I'm going to take a bath and read a good book and forget about it!"

"It's eight p.m., and I'm spending my precious free time analyzing my work situation! I'm going to enjoy this beautiful night and take my dog for a walk before bed."

"I'm feeling blue, so I'm going to work in the garden. That always cheers me up."

If you feel that you tend to get stuck in your own thoughts, here's my suggestion: Give yourself a time limit to think about something and set a timer. Check in with yourself when the timer rings and ask yourself honestly, "Am I making any progress in solving this problem?"

If the answer is "no," say to yourself—aloud if necessary—"I can come back to this later." Then go do something else that will distract you from your thoughts. If you find this difficult, make a list of good "distractors" and when you get "paralysis-analysis," look at the list. Who knows? Maybe the solution to your problem will come to you when you're busy doing something else—it often happens that way! Or maybe your problem *has* no solution, but you can feel better anyway.

Pitfall #4: Pessimism

Pessimism in this context means believing the worst-case, catastrophic scenario. If there is good evidence to think that something won't work or that danger is approaching, then by all means, take appropriate action. But when pessimism is your default response to any setback, it may be time to reframe your thoughts. Don't confuse what's possible with what's probable.

PITFALL THOUGHTS:

"I gained some weight this week—I can't make this diet work and am going to have a heart attack."

"Relationships don't work out for me, so I bet this one won't, either. I'm going to be alone forever, and then what will I do when I'm sixty?"

"I went on a job interview, but I'm sure I won't get this or any other job. What if I can't pay my mortgage next year?"

REFRAMED THOUGHTS:

"I gained some weight this week—but I haven't really given Diet Rehab a chance yet. Although it's possible that I could have a heart attack, I'm not experiencing any critical symptoms right now. I've also consulted my physician, and she said the best thing I can do for my health is lose weight."

"I'm a different person than the last time I was in a relationship, so let's see what happens now."

"I don't know whether I'll get the job or not, but I won't stop trying until I find *something* I like. Although it's possible I won't find a job for a whole year and lose the house, it's not probable. I've never gone a year without finding a job."

Pessimists are always imagining the worst-case scenario, in which any setback can easily be seen as the beginning of a catastrophe. This thinking leads to depression, anxiety, and despair. Optimists take a different approach: They imagine good possibilities that *might* happen, whether or not they ever do. Imagining these happy possibilities often gives optimists the energy to explore them, which means that optimists often end up creating good outcomes in their lives, simply because they were committed to finding a way to make the best of things or to see potential in a difficult situation. Whenever possible, they think, "Maybe it will be all right," or "I'm sure there's some good that can come from this"—and frequently, because of their positive attitude, they see possibilities to pursue that pessimists might miss.

I'm not suggesting you become a Pollyanna, blind to genuine dangers or tragedies. But I do encourage you to develop an optimistic explanatory style and that you find a way of talking yourself out of pessimistic thinking, rather than deeper into it. Creating a "can-do, can-deal-with" attitude can really help you when times are tough.

Pitfall #5: Polarization

Polarization is seeing things in terms of "either/or": black or white, yes or no, on or off. Instead of seeing that there are lots of possibilities, polarization is a pitfall in which you can only imagine "It's working" or "It's not working." That means if something isn't working perfectly, you tend to believe it isn't working at all—and probably never will.

PITFALL THOUGHTS:

"I didn't lose weight this week—my whole diet is a failure. In fact, I should go on a different diet tomorrow."

"If Terry doesn't understand this point, then this relationship is not going to work out."

"I will probably never get the respect I deserve at my current job—I obviously should quit."

REFRAMED THOUGHTS:

"I didn't lose weight this week—but I did two booster activities and feel like I made some healthy choices. I think I'm taking baby steps and making progress, even though I have a long way to go."

"Terry and I clearly see things differently when it comes to this. But we do usually agree on things. Maybe this is going to have to be an 'agree to disagree' situation."

"I think I could do more to earn respect at my job—perhaps I'll find ways to seek out additional responsibilities or have a well-timed conversation with my boss next week."

Giving up polarization does not mean that you stop taking negative factors into account. It means that you put them in context. When we're trying to make lots of changes, we often take two steps forward and one step backward, or sometimes even one step forward and *two* steps backward. Seeing the situation in a polarized way means we're far too excited about the progress—and then far too disappointed when we take that backward step. If we can reframe our thinking to accommodate all the different possibilities, we can operate on a more even keel.

Pitfall #6: Psychic

This is the frame of mind in which we're sure we know what another person is thinking, we believe *he or she* should know what *we're* thinking and what we need, and we also think we know the future. In other words, we are *sure* of a lot of things that we actually can't really know.

PITFALL THOUGHTS:

"If he cared about me, he'd see I was struggling and help me by eating healthy foods with me."

"She's not going to understand why I can't bring dessert to the party."

"I know if I go, everyone will be thinking how fat I am."

REFRAMED THOUGHTS:

"I'm going to tell him just how hard this really is for me, and I bet if I asked him to support me by trying a few booster foods, too, he would."

"She may or may not understand, but let me try explaining it to her and asking for her support—she might surprise me!"

"I feel self-conscious, but I have no idea what other people are thinking about me or even if they're thinking about me at all."

Giving up our "psychic" pitfall thinking can be very difficult because it often feels as though we're giving up our claim to know the truth and to protect ourselves. Sometimes our instincts are right on target and we have to listen to them; sometimes another person has hurt or disappointed us repeatedly, and we have to protect ourselves from trusting them again.

Sometimes, though, we're just living inside our own fears, wishes, and projections, and what we "know" is not the truth at all but merely a story we've imagined. Being rigorous with yourself about what you know and don't know—or at least about being open to the possibility that you might not know—is a good antidote for this "psychic" pitfall. Committing to telling other people what we'd like them to do in positive and specific language—as opposed to telling them what they're *not* doing in vague terms—is another good reframing device.

Pitfall #7: Permanence

Another name for this pitfall is "using the past or present to judge the future." I personally struggle a lot with this one. If I try something a few times and it doesn't work out, I have a hard time believing that it will *ever* work out, even when logic and rationality tell me that I'm giving up way too soon. I'm also prone to think, "I've always been this way—I can't change," even though I have the privilege to watch people's transformations every single day in my practice. Permanence also makes us feel like the bad way we're currently feeling will *always* be the way we feel—which becomes a self-fulfilling prophecy, because we're less likely to take action that will create change.

PITFALL THOUGHTS:

"I've never been able to lose weight, so I'm just doomed to be fat forever."

"I feel so sad and lonely. I'm always going to feel like this."

"I've never had a management job—I'm just not that kind of person."

REFRAMED THOUGHTS:

"Although I've never lost weight before, I've found a new approach to eating that just might work."

"Even though I feel sad and lonely right now, I'm doing things to change it. I remember feeling this way ten years ago, and even though things looked just as bad then, I did get out of that funk."

"I don't know if I want a management job—but it might be fun to see if some of my inherent strengths combined with learning new skills may make me a terrific manager."

It's very tempting to judge the future by the past, especially because that makes us the expert. We *know* what happened in the past, so now we can *know* what's going to happen in the future. We can protect ourselves from disappointment and maybe even avoid the hard work of transformation and growth.

I urge you to resist the lure of the "permanence" pitfall. Instead, accept that the future is unknown and that you have both the opportunity and the responsibility to create the life you want.

Booster Attributes: The 7 Ps to Master

Just as pitfall thoughts erode your brain chemistry, booster qualities *improve* your brain chemistry. In fact, the more of these booster attributes you fill your life with, the fewer pitfall thoughts you will have. All of the booster activities actually target one or more of these booster attributes, so by the end of twenty-eight days, you will look back and realize your serotonin or dopamine booster activities have created a life rich with these seven booster attributes. It's also easier to sustain booster qualities when you have sufficient serotonin and dopamine—a nice example of an *upward* spiral!

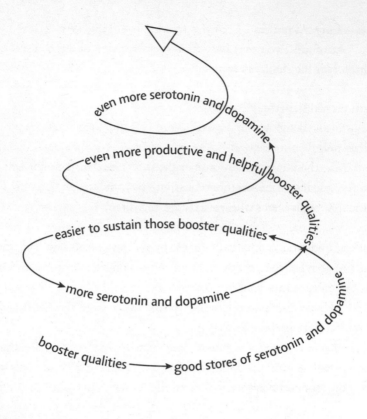

even more serotonin and dopamine

even more productive and helpful booster qualities

easier to sustain those booster qualities

more serotonin and dopamine

booster qualities → good stores of serotonin and dopamine

Here are the seven booster attributes:

Booster Attribute #1: Purpose

Filling our lives with purpose is the best way to cultivate lasting and meaningful happiness. Why are you here? What's your life's purpose on this planet? What do you think you'll remember most when you're looking back on your life? My guess is that you'll remember your relationships, the times you made a difference in the world—even on a small scale—and the work you did, paid or unpaid, that was your chance to express yourself. These things have the greatest impact on your well-being and lasting happiness. They are also the behaviors that give you lasting surges of serotonin and dopamine. If you can switch from asking "What do I want out of life?" to asking "What does life want out of me?" you may be surprised at how rich and full of possibilities your life suddenly seems.

Booster Attribute #2: Peace

What fills your life with a sense of peace or calm? And what spiritual beliefs help you to make sense of your life? As you think about the answers to these questions, consider the practices that are both spiritual *and* good for your serotonin: meditation, yoga, prayer, listening to music. Filling our lives with peace also has a direct effect on weight. A lack of peace increases the stress hormone cortisol in the brain, which tells the body to store fat in the most dangerous place—the belly. So find the activity, the pet, the relationship—and the food—that help you bring peace into your life.

Booster Attribute #3: Pride

If someone were to ask you, "What are the three things in your life that you are most proud of?" what would your answer be? When you can feel good about these answers, your serotonin and dopamine stores will rise. Enjoy the qualities and achievements that you are most proud of—revel in them and share them with others—and your brain chemistry and your waistline will benefit.

Booster Attribute #4: Power

What gives you a sense of power in your life? People who don't feel power are prone to hopelessness, anger, low self-worth, and sadness. We all need to feel powerful, to experience a sense of competency and mastery in one or more areas, throughout our lives. You can increase your sense of power by knowing you are a good parent or that you are really good at Sudoku. You can know you're a good driver, and when you use that skill to volunteer for a Meals On Wheels program, well, then you really have a double whammy in feeling good. Your serotonin and dopamine levels rise and you feel empowered, too, to make changes in your diet and your health. But if you don't think you're good at *any-thing*, then everything becomes harder. Ask yourself, "What are my strengths and how can I best use them?" In that answer lies your power.

Booster Attribute #5: Passion

What are the things in this world that truly interest you? You usually know it by your perception of time: When you're engaged in an activity you're passionate about, time seems to fly by. No two people are alike, so it's important to fill your life with things that are captivating to *you*. When we operate from this approach, our lives feel more fulfilling. We actually *want to* read up about a topic or spend our time with that hobby. You can find passion in many places—work, relationships, hobbies, or volunteer opportunities. What happens when we have more passion in our lives? You guessed it: hefty doses of dopamine in the brain, since engaging in activities you're passionate about is rewarding.

Booster Attribute #6: Productivity

One of the best things we can do when we feel sad is to distract ourselves with something that makes us feel productive. Clean out that junk drawer. Go to work. Do the laundry. Even if you don't feel like it . . . *especially* when you don't feel like it. This sort of redirection helps to decrease many pitfalls in our life, particularly paralysis-analysis, pervasiveness, and pessimism. It, too, builds our brain chemistry as it helps us to take action in our lives and instill a sense of purpose. Our serotonin increases, because we actually have more positive things to focus on.

Booster Attribute #7: Pleasure

Pleasure, dopamine, and serotonin go together like ice cream and hot fudge—or like berries and Greek yogurt. So when you're sad, get a massage! Watch your favorite TV show. Laugh. All of these are great serotonin and dopamine boosters, and maybe just the thing you need to feel good. But, remember, a truly happy and healthy life has a balance of all these boosters—so don't get stuck living a life of just pleasure!

Fine-Tuning Your Brain Chemistry

Now that you understand the basic principles of Diet Rehab, it's time to get specific. Let's move on to Part II, where you'll find out which of your brain chemicals need boosting and exactly what you need to do to boost them.

Your Brain on Food

4

Feeling Anxious: Hungry for Serotonin

A s we saw in Part I, serotonin is a key brain chemical that's crucial for many mental and physical functions. This peace-giving substance soothes, comforts, and encourages. High levels of serotonin make us feel optimistic and hopeful about achieving our goals and triumphing over our challenges. Low stores of serotonin make us feel anxious, fearful, and pessimistic about what we can accomplish.

Serotonin's importance to our brains is best illustrated by the cases of people with severely low levels. People with a history of aggressive behavior such as arson, assault, and murder have been found to suffer from drastically low serotonin levels. Self-directed violence, including self-mutilation and suicide, has also been associated with low serotonin. On a less extreme level, low serotonin has been linked to obsessive-compulsive behavior, chronic pain, chronic digestive problems, some types of sexual problems, alcoholism, sleep disturbances, chronic fatigue syndrome, migraines, cluster headaches, and eating disorders.

So when you're feeling anxious, upset, or despairing—especially when you're hungry—this is not a sign of poor character or emotional weakness. You are experiencing your body's desperate need for serotonin. The solution is not to berate, restrict, or question yourself. The solution is to feed yourself! Your body, mind, and spirit will all benefit from the booster foods and activities that you'll add when you follow the 28-day plan of Diet Rehab. And you'll be amazed that, maybe for the first time in your life, you no longer feel hungry, but full, content, and at peace.

Are You Hungry for Serotonin?

In my personal and my clinical observation, the vast majority of people in the United States are serotonin-deprived, which is why sweet, starchy foods have such a hold on us. Speaking as the kid who grew up medicating my own anxieties with ramen and full-sugar soda, I understand! Our culture is fast-paced, and our obsession with following mostly frightening or disturbing news all day long only feeds the uncertainty that most of us feel. People are much more likely to live alone than in decades past, and this can lead to increased feelings of loneliness. A working parent may feel held hostage by constant worry—especially if he or she is the only parent actively involved in the child's life. But there is a solution.

The first step in solving the problem is identifying the problem. If we can find out what is missing from your life, then we can also figure out what we need to add to your life, so you can get the serenity, hope, and peace you deeply crave. Once we target these underlying emotional issues through booster foods and activities, you may be relieved to discover that your battle with food no longer feels like a constant struggle. So let's take that first step and find out what's going on with your brain chemistry. Take the following quiz to find out whether you, too, are hungry for serotonin.

Get the Full Picture

Whatever your results, please don't stop here. You might also be ravenous for dopamine. Whether you score high or low on the serotonin quiz, check out Chapter 5 to make sure you've gotten the fullest possible picture. You need both scores to choose the version of Diet Rehab that is perfect for *you*.

Are You Hungry for Serotonin? A Quiz
Score the following:

0—never
1—rarely
2—sometimes
3—frequently
4—always

1. I feel that I'm not getting enough of one or more of the following: calm, serenity, peace, or quiet.
2. When I feel blue, my idea of comfort might include one or more of the following: cuddling, seeing a therapist, meditation, yoga, a gentle stroll, a romantic movie, peaceful music, or talking to someone to cheer me up.
3. I crave tea, wine, cigarettes, or cigars.
4. When I'm in a bad mood I crave sugar, carbs, foods with a soothing texture, such as ice cream, or soothing temperatures, such as soup, or familiar foods.
5. I don't like it when things are out of place.
6. I don't like it when people are late.
7. I question myself and wonder whether I'll be good enough to reach my goals.

8. I wonder why other people seem to have it so much more together than I do.

9. I feel lonely.

10. I prefer a job where there is not much pressure or where I can work alone without competition or demands.

11. I like to take care of others by cooking.

12. I will eat when others do, just to be polite.

13. I startle easily or am easily frightened.

14. I get stuck in anxious thoughts.

15. I'm fearful.

16. I carry tension in my body, especially my neck, back, shoulders, around the temples, or in my jaw.

17. I get headaches.

18. When I have a physical symptom, I worry about what potentially life-threatening disease I might have.

19. I have trouble falling asleep.

20. I don't like to sit still. I either pace, do something with my hands, or have something in my mouth. I rely on gum, toothpicks, cigarettes, candy, playing with my hair, or some other way of keeping busy.

21. I feel nervous.

22. I have the general feeling that things are not going to be okay.

23. I eat to calm myself down.

24. I feel overwhelmed.

25. I don't like change.

26. I consider myself a conflict-avoider or people-pleaser.

27. When things are bad, I have trouble seeing any hopeful possibilities.

28. I use sedating prescription drugs (e.g., painkillers, tranquilizers, or anti-anxiety medication) in a way I know a physician did not intend or use illegal sedating drugs (e.g., marijuana, Ecstasy, heroin).

29. I have a history of anxiety, bipolar disorder, panic attacks, obsessive-compulsive disorder, anorexia, agoraphobia, or specific phobias. (If no, score this item 0; if yes, score this item 4.)

30. I have responded favorably to anti-anxiety medication, sleeping pills, or the following antidepressants or their generic formulations: Buspar, Celexa, Cipralex, Cymbalta, Effexor, Lexapro, Lustrol, Luvox, Paxil, Pristiq, Prozac, Remeron, Sarafem, Seroxat, Serzone, Zoloft. (If no, score this item 0; if yes, score this item 4.)

SCORING

Add up your scores for items 28, 29, and 30.

Total (from boxes 28, 29, and 30 only): _____

Now, multiply this number by 3.

X3 = _____ (A)

Add up your scores for items 1–27.

Total: _____ (B)

If you are a woman, put a 5 in box C.
If you are a man, put a 0 in box C.

_____ (C)

A + B + C = _____ (D)

Your score: _____

Did Just Taking This Quiz Make You Feel Anxious?

If it did, don't worry. That's a perfectly normal reaction—especially if you're starved for serotonin—and it doesn't actually mean that anything's wrong. It only means that your default reaction to stress is to feel anxious.

The good news is that whatever your score, there is something you can do about it—something that won't be difficult and that might even be fun. Remember, *gradual detox* means that you get to keep eating everything you already enjoy while adding serotonin boosters to your diet and your life. Adding these new foods and activities will go a long way toward calming your anxieties and making you feel great. So take a slow deep breath, release it slowly, and then read on to find your score.

ARE YOU HUNGRY FOR SEROTONIN? YOUR SCORE

0–20: SATISFIED AND AT PEACE

Congratulations! Your serotonin levels are healthy, and you've figured out how to keep them that way. Your balanced brain chemistry is paying off with a feeling of well-being, self-confidence, and peace. Read the rest of this chapter to understand how you can identify your mantra and other key elements of Diet Rehab. Then move on to Chapter 5 to explore whether you are ravenous for dopamine.

21–40: HUNGRY FOR SEROTONIN: MODERATE, FREQUENT ANXIETY

If you scored in this range, your anxiety is under control, but it's a far greater presence in your life than it needs to be. You may be aware of your anxiety as something that impedes your pleasure, or you might be so used to feeling anxious that you don't even think about wanting to feel less so. (It took me a long time even to identify that I *was* anxious—I thought I was just being realistic about how scary the world was and how hard I had to work not to fail my family or to be a bad person.) Again, the good news is that you can start taking steps to make yourself feel better by undergoing gradual detox from the foods and thought patterns that are contributing to your anxiety. Read on through the rest of this chapter to find out more.

OVER 40: FAMISHED FOR SEROTONIN: MODERATE
TO INTENSE ANXIETY, ALMOST ALWAYS

If your score was over 40, your serotonin levels have fallen very low, and you are understandably desperate to feed them. You probably experience frequent, intense cravings for sugar and starch, and you may also struggle with mood swings that are linked to when and how you eat. You may be frustrated, discouraged, or despairing about how out of control you feel, both of your moods and your appetite. Please don't berate yourself any longer. You are simply doing your best to feed your brain chemistry, but you haven't yet been given the tools to help you do it effectively. Now you have those tools: Diet Rehab and gradual detox will help you rebalance your brain chemistry without making you feel deprived. Congratulate yourself for finding this book and read on through this chapter for concrete, specific suggestions that will start you on your healing journey.

Note: If you scored anything but a 0 in box A, I recommend that you work with a psychiatrist or psychotherapist to implement Diet Rehab. Your treatment may need to be augmented by medication and/or professional support.

If you scored 40 or above, please consult a psychiatrist or psychotherapist immediately to be screened and/or treated for depression, anxiety, addiction, eating disorders, or ADHD before starting this program.

> ## Do You Have Obsessive-Compulsive Disorder?
>
> One extreme presentation of serotonin starvation is obsessive-compulsive disorder. OCD symptoms include repetitive counting, obsessive checking or cleaning rituals, extremely specific rules about food, or other problematic compulsions. If you see yourself in this portrait, consult a psychiatrist before starting Diet Rehab. You may need a serotonin-boosting drug such as Luvox or Prozac; they have often been found helpful to OCD sufferers.

Serotonin and Your Body

If you've just found out that you're serotonin deficient, you might begin to see what has perhaps been behind a host of issues you've struggled with. Low serotonin causes emotional ailments such as anxiety, depression, and lack of self-confidence. It can also cause such physical disturbances as trouble with sleep, digestion, and pain. Serotonin is crucial not just for our brains but for our entire bodies.

For example, together with melatonin, serotonin is central to our ability to fall asleep, to stay asleep, and to sleep deeply. We often crave sweets or carbs late at night, which may be our body's way of seeking the natural sleep assistance of this crucial brain chemical. The problem is that the same sweets and carbs that help us fall asleep work the same way that drinking alcohol before bed does. Both may cause drowsiness, but in the long run, they actually prevent you from getting the deep sleep you need to feel rested and alert the next day. They can help you *fall* asleep, but using these foods as your sleeping aid may also lead you to wake up in the middle of the night when the "high" wears off. Healthy, stable supplies of serotonin are crucial for good sleep.

Serotonin is also active in our cardiovascular system and regulates expansion and contraction of blood vessels while also managing the function of platelets, which help blood to coagulate and close a wound. Low serotonin is implicated in Raynaud's disease and hypertension.

Digestion relies on serotonin, much of which is manufactured in the gut. Serotonin helps our abdominal muscles contract so they can push food through the gastrointestinal tract. Low serotonin may be associated with a variety of digestive problems, including irritable bowel syndrome.

Finally, serotonin is a known pain reliever. That's why when our levels are low we often feel achy and more easily laid low by any type of physical challenge. This is also why serotonin-boosting antidepressants are sometimes prescribed for chronic pain, even if the patient doesn't report depression.

I don't want you to worry about these potential maladies, but I do want you to understand: If your stores of serotonin are low, it is very difficult for you to function in a healthy, relaxed way. Eating sweet, starchy foods is an understandable response to this uncomfortable state. Unfortunately, if you try to feed your serotonin-starved brain with processed sugar and white flour, you'll only make the problem worse. First, because of the tolerance element in addiction, you'll need more and more sweet foods just to get the same comfort.

Second, because of withdrawal, you'll feel terrible any time you try to give up sugar. You reached for addictive foods in the first place because you thought they would make you feel better—and they do, temporarily. But they also conspire to make you feel worse, particularly when you are holding on to or gaining weight.

What's the solution? First, add healthy serotonin boosters to your diet and your life. Then, gradually, when you're getting all the serotonin you need, you can slowly reduce the number of pitfall foods that you were once relying on as a serotonin crutch. At the same time, as we'll see in this chapter, you can begin to replace pitfall thoughts with boosters—positive, supportive ways of thinking that will also help your serotonin levels rise.

Sugar's Sweetness Goes Beyond Taste

The brain-stimulating effects of sugar are so addictive that mice whose ability to taste sugar had been removed still chose sugar water over regular water every time they were presented with both. Clearly, neither taste nor "psychology" were involved. The mice were responding purely to the chemical effects of sugar.

Sleep, Serotonin, and Insulin Resistance: How Sugar and Carbs Make You Tired and Hungry

As we have seen, sweet, starchy foods toy with you like a seductive, unreliable lover. One minute, they're promising to satisfy all your cravings. The next minute, they've left you hungrier than ever.

The reason for this roller-coaster appetite is insulin resistance. Insulin is a hormone made in your pancreas that transfers glucose—blood sugar—from your bloodstream to your cells. We call it blood *sugar,* but that's a misleading term. Blood sugar rises or falls in response to everything you eat: proteins, vegetables, and legumes, as well as sweet or starchy foods.

However, sweets and starches cause your insulin levels to spike because processed flour and sugar metabolize quickly, dumping a lot of sugar into your blood at once. Insulin will then flood your system because it's trying to bring down those high blood-sugar levels by transferring that sugar right into your cells.

If your insulin spikes too often, your cells will eventually begin to adapt by reducing their response to insulin, which then leaves the glucose floating aimlessly in your bloodstream instead of transferring its energy to your cells. Your blood sugar is too high, and your cells aren't getting enough of it. Your pancreas will initially respond by making more insulin to saturate your insulin receptors, but over time the pancreas will start to reduce the amount of insulin it releases.

This is a recipe for diabetes and exhaustion. And most paradoxically, it also leads to a constant appetite, since your sugar-starved cells are sending hunger messages to the brain, unaware that all the sugar they need is right there in your bloodstream.

Significantly, serotonin levels rise as you eat, helping your brain to register when you feel satisfied. So if your brain is low on serotonin, it won't understand that you're "full," and you're likely to keep eating, even when your body has had enough. Besides making you feel anxious, low serotonin levels make you more likely to overeat and less likely to feel satisfied. That's why you often crave dessert, even when you feel "stuffed" and understand intellectually that you are no longer hungry. And of course, we all know that lethargic feeling we get when indulging in too many carbs and sweets, commonly known as a "food coma."

Over the long term, the weight you gain from your serotonin shortage can lead to all sorts of problems; one example is sleep apnea, which in turn can lead to restless sleep and sleepiness during the daytime. Once again, you're caught in the downward spiral of using food to make up for this general feeling of low energy, even as the food you choose depletes your energy further.

The solution? Gradually replace serotonin *pitfalls*—addictive sweets and starches—with serotonin *boosters*: foods and activities that help keep your serotonin at a nice, stable level. If you don't reverse this downward spiral, you're setting yourself up for serious health problems. It's very difficult to simply feed your serotonin addiction "a little" and remain "a little" overweight. Due to the nature of tolerance, you're going to crave ever-increasing amounts of sweets and starches, and your weight—as well as all the related health risks—will continue to increase.

The good news is that if you can turn this situation around, you'll create the opposite effect. Every healthy change will give you the energy to make more changes, which will make you even healthier.

Feel-Good Brain Chemicals

Our brains are full of chemicals that keep us moving forward in our lives, energetically but calmly. To some extent, sweet and starchy foods cue the brain to make more of these vital chemicals just as they prompt serotonin production. Luckily, the healthy serotonin boosters I'll be recommending throughout this book will also increase the levels of these other brain supports:

- **Oxytocin** promotes bonding and warm feelings of connectedness. It's released during cuddling, which is part of why you often feel close to your partner after sex. It's also released during nursing and promotes mother-child bonding. It's also released when cuddling with a pet.
- **Endorphins** are natural pain relievers that also lift our spirits. Vigorous aerobic exercise releases endorphins. So do sweet foods, which is another reason you might crave them: They really do make you feel better. Fortunately, endorphins are also released by the healthy serotonin boosters we recommend in Diet Rehab.

Cigarettes and Serotonin

Smoking is addictive because of the way it boosts dopamine. But in 2004, scientists discovered that smoking also causes the brain to reduce serotonin production. So although it feels as though smoking relieves your anxiety, nicotine actually makes you *more* anxious. In fact, the reason people so frequently overeat after they quit smoking may well be because they are trying to replace the serotonin that cigarettes have depleted.

While you are smoking, the extra dopamine from the cigarettes masks the lack of serotonin. But after quitting, both dopamine and serotonin are in short supply—causing many smokers to seek sweet, starchy, or fatty pitfall foods to make up the difference.

Why Dieting Makes You Miserable—Especially If You're a Woman

Americans quickly embraced no-carbohydrate diets, and now when people want to lose weight, cutting back the carbs is usually what they try first. But doing so can dramatically affect your brain chemistry—especially if you're a woman.

MIT researchers found that carbohydrates cause the brain to release serotonin. Without enough carbohydrates to perform this crucial function, dieters become serotonin-deprived and may feel anxious, irritable, and depressed. In one study, animals deprived of tryptophan—a key amino acid used to make serotonin—became far more aggressive. Now we can see that when dieters have a similar reaction, it's not a character weakness but a biological response.

Women and those under ongoing stress may be the most at risk. Why? They may have lower levels of serotonin in the brain and process it differently than men, so they can't afford to lose even a little as the result of a change in diet. Depressed women have been shown to respond more favorably than men to antidepressants that target serotonin, suggesting that low serotonin levels are indeed a significant problem for women and one that makes ordinary diets very problematic for most.

We know that women are about twice as likely to be diagnosed with depression as men, and they're also far more likely to suffer from migraines. Low serotonin is responsible for a great deal of that discrepancy.

Whether women lack serotonin because of their inherent biology or because they face social stressors and negative conditioning that men are spared, the result is the same: Most women are at a serotonin deficit that can easily become a serious problem if either new stress or a restrictive diet further depletes their stores.

Researchers in another study found clear evidence of women's special difficulties with diets. After three weeks on a low-calorie diet, men and women had lost a similar amount of weight. However, the women were left more anxious and unhappy and far more vulnerable to mood swings than their male counterparts. Since women's ability to produce and store serotonin may be lower than men's, the restrictive diets were harder on them. If the diets had offered women alternative sources of serotonin, the women might have lost weight *and* felt better.

Do You Worry About What Others Think?

If so, you're not alone. Those of us who feel anxious—and who are hungry for serotonin—often worry about the reactions of others. At our best, this makes us sensitive, caring, agreeable, and willing to go along with other people's plans and wishes. Be careful, though, because scientists have found that being *too* agreeable may bring a heavy price—literally. A 2007 Japanese study discovered that agreeable personalities are more likely to gain weight, perhaps because they more easily succumb to other people's pressure about where, when, and how much to eat.

Meet Your Mantra: A Powerful Tool for Self-Transformation

As we've seen, low serotonin levels produce anxiety. But it works the other way, too: Anxiety and other forms of stress deplete your serotonin.

anxious thoughts ⟶ lower serotonin levels ⟶ more anxious thoughts ⟶ even lower serotonin levels ⟶ more anxious thoughts ⟶

Does the problem start with anxious thoughts or lowered brain chemistry? No doctor can pinpoint exactly how it started for you—and it doesn't really matter. Once you start on that downward spiral, you'll keep going unless you do something deliberate to interrupt it. You need to either change your thoughts or boost your serotonin levels—or both.

Serotonin booster foods can increase your serotonin levels, so if you'd like to start adding some to your diet right now, turn to page 204. As you'll see in Part IV, your 28-day Diet Rehab plan will add serotonin boosters to your diet in a more systematic way.

But there is also quite a bit you can do to replace pitfall thoughts, which generate anxiety, pessimism, and low self-confidence with booster thoughts, which generate peace, optimism, and confidence. We already saw in Chapter 3 that there are seven pitfall thought patterns and seven booster attributes that can dramatically affect your brain chemistry. There's an even more personal way to apply these insights to yourself, and that is by working with one of the most powerful thought-transforming tools I know: your *mantra*.

Your mantra is a brief but powerful statement of your core belief about yourself and the world. Booster mantras improve our brain chemistry by creating a positive, joyous, and confident approach to life. Pitfall mantras, which are negative, make us more likely to turn to addictive foods, alcohol, or drugs, thereby keeping us anxious, pessimistic, and discouraged. The more you avoid the pitfall styles of thinking you learned about in Chapter 3, and the more you add the booster attributes to your life, the easier it will be to move from a pitfall mantra to a booster one. Likewise, the more you work on transforming your mantra, the easier it will be to avoid pitfall thinking and bring booster attributes into your life.

As you saw in the Introduction, my mantra growing up was "I'll never be a good enough son to keep my family safe, but I can't stop trying"— a pitfall mantra born out of watching my family collapse in the wake of my brother's illness. This mantra drove me to self-medicate with sweet, starchy foods that I hoped would silence the feelings of inadequacy. It also compelled me to constantly seek out how other people were feeling, what they thought of me, and what I could do to make them happy or win them over.

The problem with my mantra was that it set me up for an unease that could never be silenced and therefore a hunger that could never be satisfied. Certainly I could never do enough to make my family feel okay if they were worried about my brother's life-threatening illness and his long, slow, uncertain recovery. Nor could I ever figure out how every person in my life was feeling and then do the perfect thing to make them feel good about themselves and about me. If what I needed to feel okay was for the world to become a perfectly safe place and for every person in my life to be completely happy, I was doomed to continual feelings of insecurity and inadequacy.

Self-medicating with food only makes a pitfall mantra worse and can lead to a downward spiral if the "medicine" you're choosing is an addictive pitfall food. As we've discussed, the "sugar high" is inevitably followed by a "sugar low," just as the temporary calm of noodles and white bread gives way to an anxiety and hunger that are even more intense than before. You *can* lift your mood with booster foods—whole grains, plain yogurt, berries, and other serotonin-rich foods that feed your brain in healthy, stable ways—and later on in this book we'll find out how. But I'd also like to help you get at the thoughts and feelings that exacerbate your anxiety in the first place.

The key to this is understanding your pitfall mantra and then replacing it with a more positive message. This will interrupt the cycle of anxious thoughts and free you from its downward spiral. A positive booster mantra will allow you to feel better about yourself, your life, and your future even before you've reached your healthy weight.

Sound good? Then let's get started. The first step is to identify your mantra.

Identifying Your Mantra

If you're struggling with low serotonin, your current mantra is likely to reflect anxiety, pessimism, and a lack of confidence. Here are some common "hungry for serotonin" mantras:

- Something bad is going to happen.
- If that could happen, then anything could happen.
- I'm not okay.
- If I don't do something in one exact way, something bad will happen.
- If I'm not a complete success, I'm a complete failure.
- If I don't weigh myself frequently, my weight might balloon.
- If I don't control my feelings, I'll fall apart completely.
- If I ever let anyone down, I'm a complete failure as a person.
- If others get close to me, they'll hurt me.

Do any of these sound familiar? If one of these statements perfectly describes the way you think about yourself and the world, look no further. You have found your pitfall mantra. Go right ahead to the next section to find out how this mantra affects your weight.

But if none of these statements quite hits the nail on the head, take a few moments to articulate your own personal pitfall mantra. It's worth spending a little time on this because I want you to be able to recognize this way of thinking the moment it rears its ugly head. And believe me, it will. One thing I've learned from both my own growth and that of my patients is that as soon as we start making positive changes, all the old pitfall thoughts and feelings from the past rush up to try to pull us off track. If you can recognize your pitfall mantra, you'll be far more effective at transforming it into your new booster mantra.

So grab a notebook and a pen, or sit for a moment at your computer, and write down your own personal pitfall mantra. What words do you keep hearing that make you feel anxious, unworthy, or pessimistic? Write them down, look at them for a moment, and then move on to the next section.

How Your Mantra Affects Your Weight

Your pitfall mantra might be different from mine, but they definitely share one thing in common: Each time we repeat our pitfall mantras, our serotonin levels drop.

When you're hungry for serotonin, pitfall mantras lead to anxious pitfall behaviors—and those pitfall behaviors cause serotonin levels to drop, too. Whenever we behave in a fearful, anxious way—obsessing over every bite of food or extra ounce of weight or refusing dates until we've lost those last ten pounds—we reinforce our fearful attitudes and lower our serotonin.

This interaction between brain chemistry and experience goes back to our childhoods. Say you come from a stormy, argumentative family with a father who was always exploding in rage and a mother who was known for her frequent criticisms. As a child, you may often have felt fearful and anxious, afraid that your slightest error might provoke your parents. This state of fear would have helped to "set" your serotonin at a chronically low level. These same low serotonin levels would contribute to your anxious state.

But it doesn't stop there. Your anxious feelings might then drive you to choose fearful actions such as hanging back from the other kids at school or not wanting to leave the house until your outfit is perfect. These fearful actions in turn reinforce the idea that the world is dangerous (the kids will mock you, your outfit will make you look bad)—leading you to become still more cautious. The combination of anxious thoughts and fearful behavior continue to drive down your serotonin levels. And now we have all the elements of a vicious cycle, in which attitudes, behavior, and brain chemistry all work together to keep you anxious and miserable.

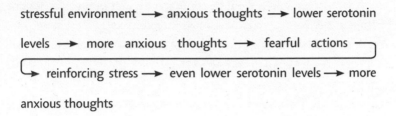

No wonder serotonin deficiency creates food addictions and weight gain! When you're feeling anxious and fearful, you're more likely to reach for the sweet, starchy foods that will ease your mind by boosting your serotonin levels. You're starving for anything that will make you feel better, and food may feel like the only comfort you can rely on.

Transforming Your Mantra

Now that you've identified your old pitfall mantra and seen how it affects your life and your weight, let's change it into a new, more positive statement about yourself and the world. For example, if your core belief is *I'm not safe*, I'm going to give you the tools to change it to a more optimistic message such as *everything is fine*. Here are some of the booster mantras you might choose:

- I'm a resourceful person and can handle the things that come up.
- Things will turn out okay . . . they usually have before.
- I'm good at many things, and if a few things aren't perfect, that's okay.
- I do what I can . . . and I'm okay with that.

- I've done my best . . . and my best is pretty good.
- Even when things are hard, I can imagine that they will get better.

Look over these improved mantras and see if one of them works for you. If so, write it down. We'll be coming back to it again later. If none of these is perfect for you, take a few moments and create your own. You deserve a booster mantra that expresses exactly the attitude and core beliefs by which you choose to shape your life.

How Diet Rehab Will Transform Your Mantra

Maya was a teenage girl who had been to three psychotherapists before me. Her parents were both attorneys who had never had a problem with their weight. Maya, on the other hand, weighed close to two hundred pounds. Her parents' high standards and fit bodies made Maya feel like a failure, as did their well-intentioned efforts to stock their kitchen with Maya's "special diet food." So when her parents weren't home, Maya would medicate her loneliness by eating boxes of cookies in the middle of the night.

Maya was a junior at a prestigious private school, where she had good friends—but no dates. She compensated for her weight by buying expensive clothes. In fact, I never saw her wear the same thing twice, and her sense of fashion was astonishing. She was also sweet, charming, funny, and incredibly smart. I knew she could have all the dates she wanted, at any weight, if she would only believe in herself and let others see her as I saw her. But I saw, too, that her mantra, "No one will ever truly love me for me," was preventing her from allowing any guy to get close. And covering up who she really was with all these accoutrements was exactly what prevented her from being seen, known, and loved.

Together we labeled all of her pitfall styles of thinking. But no amount of logical discussion was going to change the fact that no boy had ever asked her to a high school dance. Nothing we said was enough to make Maya feel pretty or love her body. And until she did feel good about herself, she would never have the stores of serotonin she needed to give up the sweets and starches that she used to medicate her misery.

"I know that logically I *should* feel good enough," Maya told me once. "That doesn't change the fact that I still *feel* sad and just awful about myself. I know I'm smart, but I keep comparing my life with other people's. Being at the top of my class doesn't really feel like it's worth very much. Honestly, if I could trade my intelligence to be sixty pounds lighter, I would. Do you know that all of my friends have kissed guys, and I actually made up this story about hooking up with a guy at camp last year? How pathetic is that? I have friends that love me, but I've never had a boyfriend. And every time I try on clothes I *feel* terrible about myself—and then nothing else that's good in my life seems to matter. My friends invite me places, but I usually just end up staying at home. I actually have been looking at colleges on the East Coast, because I just want to get away, and the idea of cold weather where I can wear heavy jackets and long sleeves all year would be such a relief to me."

What Maya was saying to me—and what perhaps you are now saying to yourself—is that words and logic aren't enough to change our feelings. In order to create a new mantra, you must give yourself new experiences. You must try out some new actions and pay attention to the consequences, and allow those consequences to affect you.

Here are a few simple examples. Do any of these speak to feelings that you recognize?

OLD BELIEF:	NEW ACTION:	NEW CONSEQUENCE:	NEW BELIEF:
I have to be perfect.	I did something imperfectly every day this week.	Nothing terrible happened.	Maybe it's okay not to be perfect *all* the time.
I am not lovable.	I smiled and said hello to a stranger five times this weekend.	Two people ignored me but three people smiled and said hello back.	Maybe there is something good in me that people can love.

The power of actions and consequences to transform core beliefs is at the heart of Diet Rehab. Signing up for a class on a topic that always intrigued you, getting in touch with old friends, treating yourself to a massage or a manicure, joining a social or political group, reaching out to ensure you have support in your life—all of these are new booster actions that will improve your brain chemistry, open you to new consequences, and allow you to really start believing your new mantra. Now we've transformed a downward spiral into an upward spiral:

booster activities ➝ positive consequences ➝ booster thoughts ➝ more serotonin ➝ more self-confidence, optimism, and peace ➝ more energy for more booster activities ➝ positive consequences ➝ *more* booster thoughts ➝ *more* serotonin

That's the payoff of Diet Rehab. Transforming and maintaining your new mantra may take a while, and you may experience some ups and downs along the way. But you can make a significant change in only twenty-eight days, and after that, the momentum of the upward spiral will help keep you on your path. Just start by adding a few booster foods and activities. Supported by a new, more positive mantra, you may be amazed at what happens next.

That's what Maya discovered. She changed the way she felt by changing her experience. After she realized that she was going to have to change her tactics to get what she wanted, she stopped being the well-dressed, funny, smart girl. Maya went to a high school party—and for once, she didn't buy a new outfit for it. She took a risk and started chatting with a guy from her math class, and instead of trying to be the funniest person in the room, she just said what she was thinking. When she told him that these parties made her feel uncomfortable, this guy blew her away by telling her that these parties made him feel that way, too. Imagine that—she wasn't the only one!

Maya was learning that what creates intimacy and connection isn't being perfect—intimacy comes from being authentic and having experiences that others can relate to. Maya and this guy ended up chatting for most of the party, and when Maya got home, she didn't feel alone. The box of cookies that she usually would have eaten stayed on the shelf.

The next day, choosing booster foods actually came pretty easily because Maya was getting more of what she was really craving in her life. When the guy from math class called to see if she wanted to hang out, she said yes. And the next night, she did something else for the first time—she ate in front of him. Maya was surprised that what she was actually hungry for was a grilled chicken salad, so that's exactly what she ate. And just like that, sustainable and gradual weight loss became possible for Maya. It had nothing to do with dieting. It had to do with her adding boosters to her life—such as connecting with somebody.

The next week, that guy became the first guy she ever kissed. Maya saw that this young man liked her just as she was, extra weight and all. And that was the ultimate booster that helped her to steadily lose sixty pounds over the next ten months. At 140 pounds, Maya still wasn't the skinniest girl in her class, but that no longer mattered to her. She had attained a healthy weight, and her life was filled with boosters like talking every day to that boy—who became her boyfriend.

Boosting Your Belief in Yourself

One of the mantra-related challenges I give my patients is the "Because . . ." exercise. I ask them to pick a positive statement about themselves that they know logically to be true and to come up with as many reasons as possible for *why* it is true. For example:

I *am* okay because:

. . . I love my mom.
. . . I'm a friendly person.
. . . My life has potential.
. . . I like where I live.
. . . My ability to sing makes me happy.
. . . I know I am a good person inside.

Sometimes I ask my patients to carry this list with them and to find at least three items to add to it throughout their day. I also ask them to reread it before every meal. These booster thoughts genuinely nourish the brain chemistry and affect how you feel and what you're hungry for. Why not give it a try? It's forcing you to put on what I call the "what's right" glasses: You're training yourself to look for the real and omnipresent evidence that supports your new mantra.

Do You Have the Happiness Gene?

Without even meeting you for a diagnosis, I can tell you the answer to this one: No. *Because there isn't one.*

Just as body weight isn't determined solely by genetics, neither is happiness. In both cases, there is an interaction between genetics, life experience, and personal choices that helps to shape our outlook as well as our bodies.

True, some of our potential for happiness *might* be contained in the levels of serotonin, dopamine, and other brain chemicals for which we are coded. Some of us are born with naturally higher ranges of those chemicals than others, and this can make a difference in our personalities, outlook, and general sense of well-being.

It's also true that our life experience affects our brain chemistry, especially during childhood. Those of us who grew up in anxious or angry households are likely to have gotten used to lower levels of key "feel-good" chemicals than people from calmer and more supportive households.

However, neither of these factors is enough to determine our destiny. As we've seen throughout this book, the decisions you make every day—choosing booster or pitfall foods, activities, and thoughts—have a profound effect on how you feel. Your biological or childhood inheritance may give you some bigger challenges to overcome, but it is absolutely within your power to create a happy, peaceful, and satisfying life.

How Cindy Changed Her Mantra

My patient Cindy had been abused since she was a child—first physically and sexually by her father, then emotionally by a series of men including two ex-husbands. Like many survivors of abuse, she had become overweight, perhaps in an effort to protect herself from unwanted attention, but also, perhaps, because her serotonin levels were low and she was almost literally starved for affection. Her mantra was "I don't deserve love, and this is how I ought to be treated."

I wanted to convince Cindy that she *did* deserve love, but I knew that this conviction could come only from within. What I could do, though, was to help strengthen the parts of Cindy that might be able to listen to and believe in this message.

When Cindy started Diet Rehab, we began by adding as many serotonin boosters as we could. Cindy knew she was free to indulge in all the sweets and starches she wanted—the sugary, soothing foods that helped her maintain her serotonin levels—but she added some new things to her diet: plain yogurt, whole-grain pasta, and chamomile tea.

I didn't want Cindy's entire focus to be on food, however, so I asked her what other treat she might give herself during Diet Rehab's first week. She thought for a while and then smiled.

"A bubble bath," she said. Cindy had loved bubble baths as a little girl, but as an adult, she'd gotten used to rushing through a morning shower. I thought that bubble baths sounded like a terrific way for Cindy to pamper herself, and the relaxing warmth of a bath sounded like a great serotonin booster as well. I suggested that Cindy splurge on seven different scents, one for each day of the week, so that she'd really commit to this nightly treat. I also asked her to take thirty seconds before and thirty seconds after each bath to say aloud the new mantra she had written for herself: "I deserve this treat, and I deserve to be loved."

Cindy felt foolish, but she agreed. When we saw each other at the end of the first week, I asked her how it had gone.

"You know how stupid I felt saying that stuff," Cindy said to me. "But by the end of the week, I don't know. Something felt different."

I thought of Cindy's response almost in mathematical terms. Before, 100 percent of Cindy believed that she didn't deserve love. Now, perhaps only 99 percent did. Cindy had accessed a tiny piece of herself—perhaps as small as 1 percent—that believed herself to be lovable and worthy. She had nurtured that part with serotonin boosters in the form of healthier foods and her special ritual. It was a small step—but it was a beginning.

During week two, Cindy added more serotonin booster activities to her life. She hated the idea of going to a gym, where she felt people would stare disapprovingly at her out-of-shape body, but she was willing to take a ten-minute walk around her neighborhood each evening. I asked her to use those walks to focus on the present moment—to notice the air on her skin, the smell of grass, the sounds of birds, the look of her neighbors' trees and lawns and gardens. This mindful walking exercise helped Cindy to immerse herself in the present moment, allowing her to take a break from listening to that negative voice inside her head. Sometimes we need to argue with our negative voices, but sometimes we just need to increase the time we spend not listening to them. Giving herself the chance to be in the "now" was Cindy's way of getting away from her pitfall mantra to just enjoy being alive.

Cindy continued adding serotonin booster foods—she was now eating fresh berries and brown rice, in addition to the yogurt, whole-grain pasta, and tea—and she continued with her nightly baths. I asked her to look at her mantra ("I deserve this treat and I deserve to be loved") at least four times a day—before and after her walk and her bath—and to jot down reasons why it was true whenever they occurred to her.

At the end of the second week, Cindy brought in the following list:

I DESERVE THIS TREAT AND I DESERVE TO BE LOVED . . .

. . . because I try to be kind to everyone in my life.

. . . because I work hard and do my best.

. . . because I am fair and honest.

. . . because I don't say mean things even when I am upset.

I was proud of Cindy for coming up with four reasons why she deserved to be loved. Just two weeks ago she couldn't think of *any*.

"But Dr Mike," she said. "I still don't *feel* like I deserve . . . anything. I wrote those things, but they were just reasons. I don't really feel them."

"I know," I said sympathetically. "But your actions are changing, and so your thoughts are changing, and pretty soon your feelings will change, too." In fact, they were already changing. Cindy looked forward to her baths and her walks. She enjoyed the taste of her new booster foods. She felt calmer and happier. Her serotonin levels were rising, and her body, mind, and spirit were feeling the difference. When I asked her how much of herself now believed her new mantra—"I deserve this treat and I deserve to be loved"—she shook her head and then said quietly, "Ten percent?"

In week 3 of Diet Rehab, we began gradually reducing Cindy's pitfall foods. Instead of several doughnuts for breakfast, she was happy to have just one, along with her yogurt and berries. Although she still had ice cream for dessert at lunch, she switched her mid-morning snack from full-sugar soda to chamomile tea. Her mid-afternoon snack was still a Danish pastry, but she was able to stop comfortably at one pastry instead of her previous two or three. She had dessert after dinner, too—sometimes pie with ice cream, sometimes chocolate cake—but instead of fries and fried chicken, she had lean grilled meats, whole grains, and some fresh vegetables. Her meals were getting healthier, her serotonin levels were rising, and she didn't feel as though she was punishing or depriving herself.

It takes at least ten exposures to a new food to accept and then enjoy it, so Cindy even found herself looking forward to the taste of some of her booster foods after a few weeks. Since it takes about four weeks to form a habit, her walks and baths were changing from obligations into normal parts of her routine.

Week 4 was transformative for Cindy. With her new, steady serotonin levels, she began to feel a sense of optimism. She could hear herself saying things like "Maybe I'll give it a try" instead of "I'm sure it will never work." Because she had been treating herself well, she was beginning to feel that other things in her life besides what she looked like gave her a sense of worth.

In this fourth week Cindy and I talked about what other activities she might like to add to her life. Cindy completely surprised both of us by saying, "I've always loved kids. Maybe I could work with them somehow." She surprised me even more by telling me that her church had a volunteer program for adults who wanted to work with troubled teens, and their next training was coming up soon.

"Is that something you want to do?" I asked her.

Cindy shook her head. "I don't know," she said in her soft voice. But the following week, Cindy let me know that she had indeed gone to the training. Before, Cindy had been so depressed about how she looked that she couldn't stand the thought of meeting strangers, but suddenly going to the meeting seemed possible. True, she spent an hour getting ready, picking out the right clothes and changing three times. But soon after she arrived at the meeting, she got to chatting with another woman around her age, and by the end of the night they had made plans to have coffee the following week.

Cindy had also begun filling her life with some of the booster attributes I shared with you in Chapter 2: in Cindy's case, passion, purpose, and pride. By stepping outside her own personal experience and helping to change other people's lives, Cindy also began to find a measure of peace.

I had encouraged Cindy not to weigh herself until day twenty-eight of her Diet Rehab. Because she had never felt hungry or deprived, she was worried that she hadn't lost weight and might even have gained. In fact, Cindy had lost nine pounds, which surprised her deeply.

"It didn't seem like I was doing much of anything," she said. When I reminded her of all the changes she had made, she shook her head once again.

"I guess each thing made the next one easier," she said. "Because the first thing I did was those baths, and that wasn't really very hard. And each thing got easier after that."

What inspired me about Cindy's story was precisely the way that each change helped support the one that came after. Each of Cindy's positive experiences reinforced her new way of looking at the world, while her booster foods and activities raised her serotonin levels, in turn increasing her confidence and her sense of self-worth. When I asked her how much of her new mantra she believed *now*, Cindy laughed.

"On a good day, about seventy-five percent," she told me. "And lately I've had a *lot* of good days." We both felt that even more improvement—in brain chemistry, attitude, and weight—was coming slowly but surely.

Satisfying Serotonin

When you begin your twenty-eight days of Diet Rehab, you'll be working to boost and balance your serotonin levels. For the first two weeks, like Cindy, you won't cut back on anything, but you will feed your body and your spirit with lots of serotonin booster foods and activities.

As you begin to make new, healthier food choices, be sure to arm yourself with information. Part of why sugar is so hard to avoid is because it's *everywhere*—even in foods you probably thought didn't have any. Sugar, high-fructose corn syrup, and other addictive sweeteners are added to bread, cereal, ketchup, fruit juices, and many other foods that you probably never thought of as "dessert." The foods you do think of as sweets may also contain far more sweetener than you imagine. A Dunkin' Donuts "Coffee Coolatta with skim milk" sounds like a healthy replacement for soda, right? After all, coffee is very low in calories and skim milk is good for you. But it actually has about the same amount of sugar as a McDonald's milk shake!

Don't let deceptive marketing sabotage your efforts to balance your serotonin. Read the labels, look up favorite fast-food treats online, and arm yourself with my booster food swap list on page 246.

When you start to feel positive reinforcement—in the form of people noticing you've lost weight, your own glances at the mirror, and your improved energy and mood—it will be easier to continue transforming your mantra into a positive and life-affirming one. Your cravings for sugar and starch will vanish, and your blood sugar will remain on an even keel. You'll feel hungry periodically, not constantly, and your food will satisfy you. And if you still desire an occasional treat— go ahead! Enjoy yourself! When your serotonin levels are high, everything about your life—including dessert—just feels better. Your mantra, your diet, and your brain chemistry will all support your going forward to create the life you were born to live.

5

Feeling Blue: Ravenous for Dopamine

When you're feeling anxious and fearful, you're hungry for serotonin. But when you're sad, lonely, or listless, you're ravenous for dopamine.

Dopamine is the brain chemical associated with thrills and challenges. When we ski down a mountain, go out on a romantic first date, or visit a foreign country for the first time, our dopamine levels rise. We feel that rush of excitement that makes life seem truly worth living.

Dopamine comes mostly from anticipation—more the thrill of the chase than the satisfaction of winning the race. It's the chemical that pushes us to seek out sex, and it's what fuels our feelings of being in love. Those first, hot six months of passion? That's dopamine. (The slower, steady warmth of a loving marriage? That's oxytocin, the "bonding chemical.") No wonder dopamine makes us feel so good!

Substances or Behaviors That Cue Our Brains to Release Dopamine

caffeine
cocaine
driving fast
falling in love
fatty foods
gambling
heroin
hunting
nicotine
red meat
risk
sex /sexual desire
shopping (not the mundane kind, but the kind known as "retail therapy")
sports, especially extreme sports
stock trading
taking risks
video games
watching an exciting sports match

Dopamine is also released with just twenty minutes of moderate exercise or eating lean protein.

When our dopamine levels are healthy, life seems fun and interesting, and we are frequently tingling with excitement. When our dopamine levels are low, we tend to feel listless and blue, trapped in a boring, dead-end life.

Lack of dopamine can also make us feel unmotivated. It becomes harder to focus on long-term goals, to defer gratification, and to muster the patience for a long, hard slog to the finish line, whether it's a project at work or a demanding emotional situation.

Low dopamine levels can send us rushing for quick-fix foods and behaviors, partly because we don't have the mental, biochemical resources we need, and we know that a high-fat treat or a stimulating behavior will give us at least temporary relief from our brain-chemistry blues. High-fat foods cue our brains to release unsustainable amounts of dopamine, giving us a chemical rush of excitement and pleasure—and setting us up for an addiction to food.

You might end up dopamine deficient for a number of reasons. Perhaps your recent life circumstances have been constricting, boring, or enervating. Lack of sleep and stress can also cause a dopamine deficiency, which is why you often crave far more when you're feeling tired or under pressure. Or maybe you're coming down from an intense, thrilling period—a passionate affair, a series of challenges, a bout of risky behavior—and you're feeling the crash. You might have inherited a tendency to lower dopamine levels or developed them through a childhood marked by high-stress and high-risk situations, such as when children grow up with a mentally ill or addict parent, or parents who are prone to rage, tantrums, or abuse. While this type of high-stress childhood can also deplete serotonin levels, it sometimes creates a kind of "roller-coaster" emotional ride for children, who get "hooked" on the adrenaline-fueled challenge of high-stakes crises, such as how to calm an out-of-control parent or how to cope with financial turmoil.

Another possibility is that, like the rats in the Scripps study, you have harmed your dopamine-pumping neurons with a high-fat diet. You may have overwhelmed your brain's ability to process the chemical, which often leads to lowered natural production.

Any type of dopamine deficiency leaves us feeling low and listless, so that we naturally turn to high-fat foods that will perk us up. Once again, we're trapped in a downward spiral:

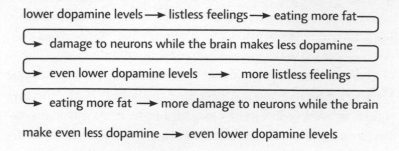

lower dopamine levels ⟶ listless feelings ⟶ eating more fat ⟶ damage to neurons while the brain makes less dopamine ⟶ even lower dopamine levels ⟶ more listless feelings ⟶ eating more fat ⟶ more damage to neurons while the brain make even less dopamine ⟶ even lower dopamine levels

In Chapter 4, we saw how low serotonin levels were connected to anxiety, pessimism, and lack of self-esteem. Low dopamine levels can lead to their own set of pitfall attitudes that soon manifest themselves in pitfall behaviors (see the chart below). Ironically, the response to both the unpleasant feelings and the upsetting behaviors often seems to be self-medication with high-fat foods. While this provides temporary relief, it also locks us even more firmly into the downward spiral.

ATTITUDES AND BEHAVIORS ASSOCIATED
WITH LOW DOPAMINE LEVELS

ATTITUDES	BEHAVIORS
depression	risky behavior
loneliness	emotional eating
feelings of being unlovable	isolating oneself
procrastination	short attention span
boredom	low sex drive
distractibility	low work performance
hyperactivity	impulsive choices

Are You Ravenous for Dopamine?

Just a quick look at the mammoth portions in U.S. restaurants should be enough to tell us that, in addition to being serotonin-starved, many of us are also dopamine-deprived. Why else would we chase high-fat foods in the form of fatty red meat, fried foods, high-fat desserts, and snacks such as crisps? Why else would we consume so much caffeine? Why else are the airwaves full of ads for energy drinks and caffeine pills? We're all exhausted, run down, and sleep-deprived—and our eating habits show it!

I have a lot of sympathy for this one, too. I look at my patients, who are often working multiple jobs or stretching themselves to the limit trying to work a full day *and* raise a family, and I can't believe how stressed they are. We're all anxious about layoffs, shutdowns, and other economic threats, and we're all under pressure to work around the clock, as well as to expend enormous energy parenting our children. Many of us are working jobs we don't enjoy or feel trapped in situations that drain us. Dopamine deficiency is the result—and craving fat, caffeine, and perhaps also sugar is the consequence.

Once again, to solve the problem, we must identify the problem. So take a closer look at your dopamine levels by taking the following quiz.

Get the Full Picture

Make sure to take both the following quiz and the one in Chapter 4 to see whether you are starving for just serotonin, just dopamine, or both. Your individualized 28-day Diet Rehab plan will depend on your own personal brain chemistry, so make sure you've gotten all the facts.

Are You Ravenous for Dopamine? A Quiz

Score the following:

0—never
1—rarely
2—sometimes
3—frequently
4—always

1. I feel that I'm not getting enough of one or more of the following: adventure, excitement, new or stimulating life experiences.
2. When I feel blue, my idea of a lift might include one or more of the following: action movies, adventure sports, loud music, screaming, hitting something, acting out, gambling, spending lots of money, or casual sex.
3. I crave coffee, energy drinks, soda, sex, cigarettes, cigars, hard liquor, or beer.
4. I crave fatty foods; foods that are new, adventurous, or spicy; or foods that have stimulating textures, such as crunchy crisps or salty popcorn, especially when I'm in a bad mood.
5. I don't mind things being out of place.
6. I often procrastinate or show up late.
7. I have gravitated toward jobs that involve risk-taking, competition, and high stakes.
8. I often find myself working with large groups of people and usually enjoy it.
9. I isolate myself and don't like reaching out when I'm in a bad mood.
10. I want things when I want them.
11. I'm not a detail-oriented person.
12. If I haven't reached my goals, that's not my fault.

13. People would say I make impulsive decisions.
14. I have trouble listening.
15. I often wonder what's wrong with other people.
16. I can't finish things.
17. I have trouble staying asleep.
18. I have lost interest in things I used to find pleasurable.
19. I like adventure and change.
20. I would rather say what I mean, even if it means hurting someone else's feelings.
21. I have trouble concentrating.
22. I feel bored.
23. I have low energy.
24. I feel restless.
25. I feel hopeless.
26. I find myself crying or tearful.
27. I feel generally dissatisfied with life.
28. I use prescription stimulants in a way I know a physician did not intend, or use illegal activating drugs (cocaine, crystal meth, speed, steroids), or ephedra/ephedrine-based workout or diet formulations.
29. I have a history of depression, bipolar disorder, or ADD/ADHD. (If no, score this item 0; if yes, score this item 4.)
30. I have favorably responded to ADD/ADHD stimulant medication, ADD/ADHD non-stimulant Strattera, or to the following antidepressants or their generics: Cymbalta, Effexor, Pristiq, Remeron, or Wellbutrin. (If no, score this item 0; if yes, score this item 4.)

SCORING

Add up your scores for items 28, 29, and 30.

Total (from boxes 28, 29, and 30 only): _____

Now, multiply this number by 3.

X3 = _____ **(A)**

Add up your scores for items 1–27.

Total: _____ **(B)**

If you are a man, put a 5 in box C.
If you are a woman, put a 0 in box C.

_____ **(C)**

A + B + C = _____ **(D)**

Your score: _____

Did Just Taking This Quiz Make You Feel Inadequate?

People have that reaction frequently, because—especially if you're deprived of dopamine—you may frequently feel that you're just not measuring up, can't get the job done, or don't have the internal resources to do what you would like to do.

I want to stress that this feeling is not a direct reflection of who you are or what you can achieve. Feeling inadequate is a common reaction to a dopamine shortage, and when your brain chemistry is balanced, you're likely to feel quite different. The good news is that whatever your score, there is something you can do about it—something that won't be difficult and is likely to feel good. Remember, gradual detox means that you get to keep eating all the foods you already enjoy while adding dopamine boosters to your diet and your life. These boosters will help you find the motivation to get moving, the patience to reach your goal, and the energy to get there. So shake off the sense of inadequacy, prepare yourself to take action, and read on to find your score.

ARE YOU RAVENOUS FOR DOPAMINE? YOUR SCORE

0–20: MOTIVATED AND ENERGETIC

Congratulations! Your dopamine levels are healthy, and you've figured out how to keep them that way. Your balanced brain chemistry is paying off with a feeling of excitement and pleasurable anticipation as you look forward to your life. Make sure you have thoroughly read Chapter 4 to explore whether you are hungry for serotonin. Then move on to Part III to learn how to fill your diet with foods and activities that will boost your serotonin and dopamine levels and help you keep them at a healthy level.

21–40 : RAVENOUS FOR DOPAMINE: MODERATE LISTLESSNESS, IMPATIENCE, OR SENSE OF INADEQUACY

If you scored in this range, your dopamine is at a moderately low level, and it's bringing you down. You are not as motivated as you would like to be, and you are frequently plagued with feelings such as "What's the use?," "I'm not going to make it," or "I don't see the point of even trying." You can find your energy and rediscover life's pleasures by beginning your gradual detox from the foods and thought patterns that are contributing to your listlessness. Read on through the rest of this chapter to find out more.

OVER 40: FAMISHED FOR DOPAMINE: PERSISTENT, SOMETIMES OVERWHELMING DEPRESSION, LISTLESSNESS, OR FATIGUE

If your score was over 40, your dopamine levels have dropped to a seriously low level, and you may be desperate to bring them back up. You are likely to feel intense cravings for high-fat foods, and you may also struggle with feelings of fatigue, depression, or despair that improve only temporarily when you eat or over-caffeinate. You may be worried or confused about why you can no longer access your usual energy and excitement. Please don't be concerned. Your brain chemistry has gotten out of balance and while you might be doing your best to restore its health, you perhaps don't have the right information to help you do it effectively. Now you can take action, starting with your program of gradual detox and Diet Rehab. Keep reading to find the tools you need to make an action plan.

Note: If you scored anything but a 0 in box A, I strongly recommend that you work with a psychiatrist or psychotherapist to implement Diet Rehab. Your treatment may need to be augmented by medication and/or professional support.

If you scored 40 or above, please consult a psychiatrist or psychotherapist immediately to be screened and treated for depression, anxiety, addiction, eating disorders, or ADD/ADHD before starting this program.

Dopamine Deprivation: Harder on Men?

I am living testimony to the fact that many people don't fit the gender stereotypes, which proclaim that men tend to be dopamine-deprived while women are starving for serotonin. Speaking as a man who struggles more with serotonin issues, I know that many people do *not* align with the generalizations.

Having said that, I want to acknowledge that many studies do associate women with a craving for sweets and ice cream, while men do seem to be drawn to red meat and other high-fat foods. There does seem to be some biological basis for this difference, whether we're born with it, develop it in response to cultural conditioning, or a little of both.

However it came about, adult men may produce more serotonin and store it more effectively than women do. When men and women were subjected to the same stressors during research, eight times more blood flowed to the emotional centers in women's brains than to those of the men, suggesting that women use up their serotonin reserves more quickly than men and are more easily drained by stress. Women are about twice as likely to suffer from low-serotonin depressions than men and are also more likely to be anxious, another sign of low serotonin. Some studies show that women respond better to the antidepressants that target serotonin, suggesting that their problems lie in low serotonin levels, and their problems are eased when their serotonin levels are boosted.

Men, on the other hand, seem to be more hooked on dopamine. A 2006 study found that men are more susceptible to the effects of drugs that actively affect dopamine levels. When both men and women were given doses of amphetamines, the men's brains were flooded with far more dopamine than the women's. Men are also much more likely to be diagnosed with ADD/ADHD, also associated with low dopamine.

Some researchers speculate that men are responding to a uniquely male gene that regulates their brains' production of dopamine. Perhaps this is why men are more likely than women to develop such dopamine-related diseases as schizophrenia and Parkinson's, a condition in which dopamine-producing neurons in the back of the brain begin to die, producing the body tremors and paralysis that indicate a lack of that neurochemical.

The Dopamine Reward

If you're struggling with low dopamine, you may also have noticed a subtle way that dopamine itself acts to keep all types of addictions going. Any time we feel a sense of pleasure or the satisfaction of a craving, we get a little dopamine kick. This is true whether we're craving serotonin, dopamine, or any other brain chemical—or whether we're craving a person, an experience, an object, or a substance. Dopamine gives us a potent reward that makes it even harder to resist our cravings.

At the same time, if our dopamine levels are too low, we don't get the kick we seek from the high-fat food we turned to—and so we may continue craving fat until our dopamine levels finally rise. This relationship emerged in one study when researchers asked groups of young women to drink a milk shake while they monitored the effects it had on their dopamine levels. The women whose brain activity showed the lowest dopamine levels in the study were most likely to have gained weight when researchers met them a year later. Researchers speculated that if a woman's dopamine levels were relatively low even after a delicious milk shake, she was more likely to crave fatty foods in other instances.

What does this mean for you? If you're trying to overcome a craving for dopamine, be extra compassionate with yourself, because it may feel as though your entire body is conspiring to pull you back into the addiction. Since dopamine itself is the reward for any type of pleasure—whether satisfying an addiction or something healthier—it's hard not to want more and more and more of it. That's why I want you to be especially careful to load up your diet and your life with dopamine boosters while you are trying to let go of the unhealthy choices that are making you feel both bad and good.

ADHD and Dopamine

Many studies have linked dopamine to attention-deficit hyperactivity disorder (ADD/ADHD). In a recent study that involved performing brain scans on people with ADD/ADHD who had never taken medication for the condition, the scans revealed dopamine levels that were significantly lower than normal. This makes sense, because the medications used to treat

ADD/ADHD, including the antidepressant Wellbutrin and stimulants such as Adderall and Concerta, all increase dopamine levels in the brain.

Other studies have suggested that ADD/ADHD sufferers are more vulnerable to other types of addiction because they are unconsciously self-medicating, desperately trying to increase their low dopamine levels the only way they know how.

Paying the Price for Your Caffeine Buzz

A key dopamine stimulator is caffeine, which some 90 percent of all U.S. adults consume daily, primarily in the form of coffee, energy drinks, and soda. Like sugar, starches, and fats, caffeine gives us a quick high followed by an uncomfortable crash. In many cases, our response to that crash is to seek either high-carb or high-fat foods to pick us up again. While caffeine does suppress your appetite during the buzz, you might feel hungrier than ever when you crash.

Lack of sleep lowers both your dopamine and your serotonin levels. Caffeine can also interfere with your ability to get restful sleep—and that lack of rest lowers both your dopamine and your serotonin levels. If you're already getting less sleep than you need—and most Americans are—you may be turning to a combination of sweet, starchy, and high-fat foods plus various forms of caffeine just to make it through the day.

What's the solution? First, get more sleep—easier said than done, I know, but crucial to your health, well-being, and weight loss. Besides decreasing your levels of vital brain chemicals and setting you up for food cravings, lack of sleep increases the production of cortisol, which, as we saw in Chapter 1, cues your body to hold on to fat.

Second, take a long, hard look at how caffeine might be affecting your rest. The half-life of caffeine is six hours, which means that the coffee or energy drink you consume at four p.m. is leaving you with a half-dose of caffeine by ten p.m. Even when you have no problems falling asleep, caffeine interferes with the depth of your rest. If you wake up the next day feeling tired, you're setting yourself up to crave more caffeine—and then all the sugar, starch, and fat that helps you through your caffeine cycle.

Of course, if you're drinking any of the delicious flavored coffee drinks that are so popular these days, you are most likely adding sweets and fats to your caffeine anyway. This combination makes these treats especially hard to resist—and also especially likely to set you up for addiction, exhaustion, mood swings, and weight gain.

In your 28-day Diet Rehab plan, I'll include suggestions for reducing pitfall levels of caffeine, whether in the form of coffee, soda, or energy drinks. Remember, I won't ask you to cut back on anything—not even a little bit!—until you've spent two entire weeks boosting your dopamine and serotonin levels with foods and activities that will give you some of the same lift that caffeine does now. If just the thought of cutting back the caffeine makes you anxious, please put it out of your mind. You won't be trying to do without your caffeine buzz until you're getting that same kick elsewhere—I promise!

Why Diet Soda Is Bad for Your Waistline

Okay, I used to be a soda junkie, so I know how awful this next sentence is going to sound, but I have to be straight with you, so here it is: Diet soda interferes with your weight loss.

Why? Because it's so sweet that once you develop a taste for it, nothing tastes sweet enough anymore. Your palate will have a very hard time preferring a sweet, delicious apple over a diet soda as long as the soda option is available. So diet soda can actually keep you from choosing foods that are going to prevent disease and weight loss. It's no wonder so many studies show that people who drink diet soda are more likely to be overweight.

The good news is that you can fix this through taste recalibration. Think of it as your car needing an alignment after hitting a big pothole. After this recalibration occurs, you will actually *stop liking* the taste of that hundreds-of-times-sweeter-than-sugar taste. Just as people on a low-sodium diet eventually report previously preferred foods as too salty, the same thing can happen to your taste buds that perceive sweetness. (For more on taste recalibration, see Chapter 10.)

Again, I won't ask you to even *think* about cutting back on diet soda until your life and diet are full of serotonin and dopamine boosters. So please don't worry about it now. Just be aware that diet soda is a pitfall food, and when you're looking at your 28-day Diet Rehab plan, you'll be counting diet soda as one of your treats.

Are You Addicted to Soda?

If the very idea of cutting back on soda makes you want to run screaming for the hills, consider the possibility that you may be using its high doses of caffeine or sugar to self-medicate other concerns. In my experience, hard-core soda drinkers—diet or full-sugar—are sometimes trying to treat underlying depression or ADD/ADHD-like symptoms with dopamine-boosting caffeine, or to address underlying anxiety or low self-worth by loading up on the serotonin-boosting sugar in regular soda. Other times excessive soda/caffeine consumption means their body just needs a little more rest.

Either way, pairing these biochemical needs with a habit you've been engaging in for years can give way to an unhealthy compulsion. Luckily, Diet Rehab's dopamine booster foods and activities can help you achieve the same effect in a healthier way. Boosters such as meditation have also been shown to be clinically effective in treating ADD/ADHD, so you'll need less caffeine to feel focused.

If you're turning to caffeine because you're exhausted, serotonin boosters will help you achieve the peace you're craving. Thirty minutes of extra sleep or a ten-minute walk outside your office is another great remedy for exhaustion and stress. A Sudoku puzzle or cup of green tea may be a great replacement for soda when you need a little pick-me-up. You don't have to decrease *anything* before we start *adding* to your life.

And, remember, at no point in Diet Rehab are you ever asked to cut anything out of your diet entirely. You can always have at least a little of anything you'd really like.

So if you really want that diet soda, go for it! But I bet you'll be craving it less after you've completed the program. If you're still noticing significant symptoms, such as inability to focus, hyperactivity, depression, or anxiety, consider seeing a psychiatrist or psychotherapist.

Revving Up Your Brain—Naturally

Dopamine usually works with two other activating brain chemicals that, luckily, are also supported by our dopamine boosters: adrenaline (also known as epinephrine) and noradrenaline (also known as norepinephrine). These stress hormones are designed to rev us up for "fight or flight," and they are key elements in feeling motivated, excited, challenged, and thrilled.

People with ADD/ADHD are often treated with dopamine-boosting stimulants or Wellbutrin, an antidepressant that boosts dopamine. Sometimes, though, they are prescribed the nonstimulant Strattera, a "norepinephrine reuptake inhibitor," which basically increases the available norepinephrine in the brain. People with depression are often given a class of drugs known as SNRI—serotonin norepinephrine reuptake inhibitors— which increase both the serotonin and the norepinephrine available to the brain.

Diet Rehab is also geared to address these vital brain chemicals. If you get plenty of dopamine boosters, you will also be supporting your adrenaline (epinephrine) and noradrenaline (norepinephrine) levels as well.

Low Dopamine: Frustration, Boredom, and Feelings of Inadequacy

By now you understand that low dopamine levels create listlessness, frustration, boredom, feelings of inadequacy, and, in some cases, full-blown clinical depression. But it works the other way, too: being trapped in a frustrating, boring, or discouraging situation depletes your dopamine.

discouraged thoughts ⟶ lower dopamine levels ⟶ more

discouraged thoughts ⟶ even lower dopamine levels ⟶ more

discouraged thoughts

Which came first, the thoughts or the brain chemistry? Like the chicken and the egg, we can't pinpoint it exactly—but it doesn't matter. What does matter is interrupting your pitfall thoughts while revitalizing your brain chemistry.

Dopamine booster foods are crucial for giving you the lift that you may now be getting from caffeine, nicotine, or high-fat foods. If you want to start adding these boosters to your diet immediately, turn to page 219. When you get to Part IV, you'll learn how to craft your 28-day Diet Rehab plan and how to add dopamine boosters to your diet every day, giving you the emotional and biochemical support you need to get off the caffeine "buzz-crash" roller-coaster.

You can also harness the power of your mind to replace *pitfall* thoughts, which generate discouragement, fatigue, and lack of motivation, with *booster* thoughts, which generate excitement, energy, and determination. As we saw in Chapter 4, transforming your mantra by adding booster activities is one of the most powerful thought- and mood-transforming tools you can have.

Novelty and Obesity

Novelty-seeking personality types are more likely to crave a dopamine hit—and are also more likely to be obese, according to recent research. A 2006 study found that obese people were more likely to be novelty seekers than the control group. Since novelty seeking is also associated with impulsivity and gratification seeking, a possible explanation for the higher weight is that this personality type was more likely to give into their cravings while failing to consider long-term consequences.

Identifying Your Mantra

If you skipped Chapter 4, go back and read "Meet Your Mantra" (pages 84–91) to find out what a mantra is and how it can help you replace pitfall thoughts with booster thoughts. If you're coping with low dopamine, your mantra is likely to express discouragement, defeat, and a sense of inadequacy. Here are some common "ravenous for dopamine" mantras:

- Something has to change.
- I'm just not good enough.
- I never really succeed.
- I let people down a lot.
- My life is not going the way I thought it would.
- I can't finish anything.
- No one really understands me.
- Is this all there is?
- I just can't get started.
- I can't do anything right.
- Something's wrong with me.
- I just can't get it together.

- I feel helpless.
- I wish I was somewhere else.

I know it's not pleasant looking at such negative statements, but like a surgeon getting ready to cut out an unhealthy growth, we've got to identify the problem with precision before we can do anything about it. Every one of us tells ourselves a story about the world and who we are—a story that is embodied in our mantra. Our mantra tells us what we can expect, from the world and from ourselves. If we're going to change our behavior and get new results, we will get a lot further if we start by changing our mantra. But we can't *change* our mantra until we *identify* our mantra.

So what's *your* mantra? Do any of the ones above sum up your sense of yourself and the world? If so, this is your pitfall mantra. Write it down and then go right to the next section to find out how this mantra affects your weight.

If none of the statements I've supplied accurately describes you, now is the time to write down your own personal pitfall mantra. Take a few minutes and really get down the sentence or phrase that captures your core beliefs about who you are and how the world responds to you. What words do you keep hearing that make you feel discouraged, unmotivated, and inadequate? Please write them down somewhere you can easily access them and then proceed to the next section.

How Your Mantra Affects Your Weight

As we saw in Chapter 4, your pitfall mantra has a powerful effect on your brain chemistry. Each time you repeat it to yourself—even unconsciously—your dopamine levels fall a little bit. If you feel trapped inside these thoughts, you will feel trapped inside your life—and your brain chemistry will reflect that:

restrictive environment ⟶ angry and/or discouraged thoughts ⟶
↳ lower dopamine levels ⟶ more despair and less motivation to
change ⟶ no action, or only reckless action ⟶ more restrictions
in your life ⟶ even lower dopamine levels ⟶ more despairing
thoughts

You can easily see how dopamine deficiency creates food addictions
and weight gain. The more unmotivated and discouraged you feel, the
more you reach for the caffeine to perk you up while turning to high-fat
foods that bring you momentary pleasure. You're ravenous for a sense
of aliveness and purpose—and caffeine, fat, and perhaps risky or exciting behavior may feel like the only pleasure you can expect.

Transforming Your Mantra

Seeing how your old pitfall mantra keeps you stuck in an unsatisfying
cycle—and how it contributes to weight problems—you may now be
ready to choose a new, positive mantra to replace it. Here are some possible choices for a booster mantra:

- When I've made a real effort to communicate with people I
  love, they are willing to help me.
- There are many things I am good at, and the more I focus on
  my strengths, the better I feel.
- I am successful in many areas of my life, and weaknesses are
  opportunities for growth.
- There are many people who love me.
- My life is not exactly how I imagined it, but there are many
  things that I'm proud of and still some things I'd like to achieve.

- When I use successful strategies, I'm effective at getting things done.
- There are many things that make me happy. The emptiness I'm still feeling is information that I need to change or add something to my life.
- Here I am, and I'm going to *live* this life I was given.
- I'm here on this earth to find out what life wants out of me—not what I want out of life.

Choose a booster mantra from the list or create your own, writing down exactly the phrase that expresses how you would like to see yourself and the world. We'll come back to it again later, so I'd like you to have it ready. The right booster mantra can be a powerful tool in shaping your life, not to mention your body, and I want you to choose one that you feel perfectly articulates the self and the life you want.

Using Diet Rehab to Transform Your Mantra

As we saw in Chapter 4 (pages 71–100), changing your mantra is not necessarily a simple task. No matter how often you tell yourself that you *should* feel different about yourself, the fact remains that you feel the way you feel. If you're discouraged, unmotivated, or depressed, then those are your feelings, and logic doesn't necessarily enter the picture.

However, what does change your self-concept and your mantra is *experience*. Trying out new actions and noticing the consequences allows you to re-create your life.

Check out these examples of old beliefs transformed into new. Can you relate to any of them?

OLD BELIEF:	NEW ACTION:	NEW CONSEQUENCE:	NEW BELIEF:
I'm just not good enough.	I'm going to sign up for that Spanish class I've been thinking about.	I realized I'm quite good at learning foreign languages. I'm a smart person.	I'm good at many things.
Something has to change.	I'm going to list the three things I'm most grateful for, and I'm going to spend ten minutes writing about the one area in my life I most want to change.	I feel happy acknowledging all that is right in my life. And when I was really honest with myself, I realized that I'm not feeling fulfilled in my work. I'm going to go to that open house at the university to see if their programs could be an option for the long term.	Life is full of opportunities to grow and change.

Taking action to create new experiences is what makes Diet Rehab effective. Going on a trip to a place you've never been, challenging yourself with puzzles and brain teasers, trying out different types of food, exploring a new hobby or a new form of exercise—all of these are dopamine booster actions that will allow you to see fresh possibilities, in both your life and yourself. That's how to change a downward spiral into an upward spiral:

booster activities ➝ positive consequences ➝ booster thoughts ➝ more dopamine ➝ more excitement, vitality, and motivation ➝ more energy for more booster activities ➝ positive consequences ➝ *more* booster thoughts ➝ *more* dopamine

You won't necessarily be able to change everything overnight. But you can make small changes that you'll feel right away. Over time, step by step, change by change, you'll discover that you've created a new mantra—and a new life. The first step is simple: Add a few booster foods and activities to your diet and your life. After that, who knows?

Supporting Your New Mantra

As we saw in Chapter 4, I always ask my patients to create support for their new mantras by giving reasons why they're true (see page 93). Here's an example of how that might work for a dopamine-boosting mantra:

I am successful in many areas of my life . . .

because I try hard.
because I am talented at what I do.
because of who I am.
because when given a challenge, I rise to it.

Jim's New Mantra: Losing Weight, Gaining Zest

Jim was a good-looking thirty-nine-year-old guy who loved to hit the bars most nights after work, where he'd hang out with his buddies and chat with women. He was proud of his ability to score, and usually went home with a different woman a few times a week. He lived on pizza and burgers and never cooked for himself, relying on smoking to curb his appetite and keep his weight under control.

Lately, though, he noticed that he'd been gaining weight. He'd also been trying to quit smoking, unsuccessfully, and it was the frustration with both situations that pushed him to seek psychotherapy with me.

"I try to stop smoking," he told me, "but three days is the most I've ever gone without a cigarette. I just feel desperate and like I can't get anything done if I'm not smoking."

"What do you do when you're *not* smoking?" I asked him.

Jim laughed, bitterly. "Mostly, I just eat," he said. "It's kind of out of control. The other day I had pizza for breakfast and then a huge plate of chili cheese fries for lunch. I've always been a big eater, but this is getting ridiculous."

Eventually, Jim told me that he was becoming dissatisfied with other aspects of his life. Picking up women—though he still felt successful in that regard—had lost a lot of its appeal. He was tired of spending time with women he didn't really like, who either wanted more than he felt like giving or whose lack of interest made him feel even less satisfied with the routine sex. His job as an advertising salesman required him to be constantly charming, peppy, and "up." But, Jim told me, "Nobody really cares about me. They just want to know what I can do for them."

Jim had seen himself as a wild man, a daring rebel who played by his own rules. He'd spent a lot of time pursuing extreme sports when he was younger and had broken some bones skateboarding and playing rugby. In his twenties, he'd had the energy to be physically active even though he smoke, drank, and got little sleep. Now he felt as though everything was catching up with him and he wondered what the point was. As he sat before me in my office, I saw a depressed, overweight, and lonely man with no energy, motivation, or zest for life.

Together, Jim and I agreed to embark on a 28-day Diet Rehab program that was designed to boost his dopamine levels with healthy, sustainable choices so that he could let go of smoking, get his drinking under control, and lose the weight that was making him feel bloated, lethargic, and unattractive. I explained that we needed to "reboot" his natural production of dopamine, which I believed was severely impaired by his lifelong high-fat diet.

For the first two weeks of Diet Rehab, I told Jim to smoke and drink as much as he usually did, and to eat all the same high-fat foods he craved. But I also had him add a few new dopamine booster foods each week: lots of lean meats and fish, some celery sticks with salsa, a few servings of dark green, leafy vegetables, some sweet peppers. To increase his motivation, I had him check out my booster food swap list and a few booster recipes, so he could still have pizza and burgers but without gaining weight because *most* of his food would be coming from healthier sources.

I also encouraged Jim to add some dopamine booster activities to his life. Because Jim felt so listless and unmotivated, he didn't really feel like starting anything new, but after some brainstorming, he realized he might enjoy Sudoku. He carried a book of puzzles with him that first week and found the mild challenge to be pleasantly stimulating.

The second week of Diet Rehab, Jim was looking for another dopamine booster activity, and he remembered that he used to be interested in hiking. Reluctantly, he joined a local hiking club and forced himself to get up early one weekend morning for a brisk walk through the mountains. Almost against his will, he enjoyed himself—partly because he met a woman who, he told me, "Is the first girl I've been excited about in a long, long time." The woman in question had just come out of a messy divorce and wasn't eager to get involved. For Jim, the challenge of wooing and winning her over proved to be just the dopamine booster activity he'd been looking for, besides giving him motivation to continue with the next two weeks of Diet Rehab.

A few months after Jim's first twenty-eight days of Diet Rehab, Jim finally accepted that this woman wasn't really for him. But by then he'd lost a lot of the weight he'd wanted to let go of, developed a new interest in hiking, and shifted his food choices. He still loved burgers and pizza, but he wasn't eating them compulsively. Maybe twice a week he would have a burger and twice a week pizza. The rest of his weekly meals were far more balanced—and, now that Jim had reset his brain chemistry, they were satisfying, too.

Through the course of his twenty-eight days on Diet Rehab, Jim also worked on changing his mantra. Originally a mixture of "I'm just not good enough" and "My life isn't going the way I envisioned it," it had morphed into "There are many things I'm grateful for, and my feeling of emptiness is information inviting me to make some changes."

Jim is still struggling with what he truly wants out of life. He's re-evaluating whether he's in the right line of work, thinking about the kind of woman he'd like to be involved with, and figuring out what his life plan should be. By adding dopamine booster foods and activities to his diet and his life, he's regained his motivation. Oh, and he's also quit smoking. "For the first time in a long time," Jim told me recently, "I'm excited about the future instead of depressed by it." His words are a tribute to the power of brain chemistry—and to Jim's personal power to re-create his life.

Revitalizing Dopamine

Your goal through your twenty-eight days of Diet Rehab is to restore your body's natural production of dopamine, which will in turn restore your ability to enjoy your life. For the first two weeks, like Jim, you won't deprive yourself of anything you want, but you will simply add dopamine boosters like high-protein, low-fat foods and challenging activities. The booster foods will cue your body to make sustainable amounts of dopamine, getting you off the "buzz-crash" cycle that caffeine and high-fat foods can create. Your fat cravings will evaporate while your caffeine cravings will decrease. You'll find yourself losing weight without even trying, even as you still enjoy your favorite foods—but in moderation, not in excess. Your reward will be a renewed pleasure in all aspects of your life and renewed motivation to go forward making the choices you want.

6

Feeling Powerless: Starving for Everything

f a common serotonin deficient mantra is "I don't feel safe" and a dopamine deficient one is "I'm not good enough," the double-deficiency
mantra is "Help! My life is out of control!" If you tested low in both
categories, you may feel that both you and your life are out of control.
You may have gone through a series of stressful events—perhaps a parent's illness, the end of a relationship, a child's crisis, or difficulties at
work. You might feel that you once used to have an easy relationship
to food and eating, but that now, for the first time in your life, you
don't. Or perhaps you always struggled with your relationship to food
but now you feel it's gotten the best of you. Possibly you feel that
you've always been out of control when it came to food—and perhaps
to other life issues, too—and you're turning to Diet Rehab with the
hope that you can finally regain control and restore your sense of personal power.

What does it mean to feel out of control? Below are some possibilities. Not all the descriptions will apply to any one person; they are a

range of ways that you might feel or behave. Do you recognize yourself in any of the descriptions?

LOW SEROTONIN LEVELS	LOW DOPAMINE LEVELS	LOW LEVELS OF BOTH SEROTONIN AND DOPAMINE
ATTITUDES: anxious, fearful, helpless, pessimistic, uncertain, unconfident	**ATTITUDES:** angry, depressed, despairing, fatigued, hopeless, listless, unmotivated	**ATTITUDES:** "at the end of your rope," confused, exhausted, frantic, "frozen," hysterical, powerless
BEHAVIORS: obsessing and worrying constantly over relationships, money, work, or the future; avoiding decisions; feeling clingy, dependent, and needy; having difficulty falling asleep, often because of worry; frequent or continual craving of sweet, starchy foods	**BEHAVIORS:** flying off the handle at little things, often unexpectedly; feeling unable to do the simplest tasks; not being able to concentrate; frequently berating yourself for mistakes and reminding yourself of your inadequacies; shutting down thoughts and feelings in order to avoid feeling inadequate; possibly engaging in risky behaviors around gambling, drugs, sex, or physical risk; difficulty remaining asleep; frequent or continual craving of high-fat foods	**BEHAVIORS:** alternately reaching out to people and pushing them away; crying in a way that feels out of control; forgetting things or becoming easily confused; isolating yourself; sleeping too much or too little; generally feeling helpless and out of control; wanting sex far more often or far less often than usual; frequent or continual craving of both sweet and starchy foods and of high-fat foods

As you can see, when both your serotonin and dopamine levels are too low, you tend to crave both the sweet, starchy foods that indicate a serotonin deficiency and the high-fat foods that denote a lack of dopamine. Because your brain chemistry is so out of whack, your cravings may be even more intense than those of the person who lacks only *one* vital chemical, as might your other responses. Where someone with a mild serotonin deficit might feel a little clingy, you burst into tears when a friend says she has to get off the phone; where someone with a moderate dopamine deficiency might be irritable, you find yourself erupting in rage when your spouse forgets to buy the milk. Both your internal and your external worlds may feel beyond your control, exacerbated by your frequent or continual cravings for food and your seemingly boundless appetite.

Whether this is a familiar condition or a recent development, it's profoundly dispiriting and has led you to fall into the seven pitfall thought patterns described on page 53. You may have tried to regain control of your eating, your life, or your own responses, and if you weren't 100 percent successful, or if you couldn't maintain the control you had won, you probably felt even worse about yourself. These bad feelings depleted your stores of serotonin and dopamine still further, sending you into yet another version of a downward spiral:

recent or long-term life stress or family situation ➞ low levels

of serotonin and dopamine ➞ feeling powerless, overwhelmed,

and out of control ➞ *lower* levels of serotonin and dopamine⌐

➞ feeling even *more* powerless, overwhelmed, and out of control

If this is your situation, don't worry. The more intense, overwhelming, and out-of-control your feelings toward food have become, the more likely that a brain-chemistry imbalance is involved. That's actually good news, for two reasons: One, the problem isn't an essential one about you, your personality, or your strength of character but is rather a fixable problem that can be addressed with different food and lifestyle choices. Two, I'm offering you an approach to eating that starts by adding booster foods and activities, *not* by taking anything away. Unlike diets that have failed in the past, adding foods and activities rather than asking you to give something up is going to allow you the sustainable benefits of gradual detox. Previously, any diet was almost bound to fail because it put you into a state of withdrawal that would be especially painful for someone who was short on both serotonin and dopamine. Diet Rehab will ease you through the withdrawal period without your even realizing that it's happened. So let's get started. It's time to help you shift your mantra from "I'm out of control" to "I know my strengths and weaknesses, and I can make healthy decisions."

Rewriting Your Mantra

If necessary, review the sections on mantras in Chapters 4 and 5 (pages 84 and 118). Then identify your current pitfall mantra. Here are some possible choices:

- I can't handle anything—I'm just a mess!
- I've really screwed everything up, and I'm paying for it now.
- Why does everything in my life always go wrong?
- No matter what I try, it's just no good—and I'm getting tired of trying.
- Help! I'm out of control.

You can also write your own unique pitfall mantra, one that describes your own personal mental and emotional state.

Next, choose a new booster mantra that will support you in your efforts to restore your brain chemistry and take back your life. Here are some possible choices:

- It's time I started dealing with my problems, and with some help, I'll be able to handle them.
- There are things that have happened to me that weren't my fault, and now it's time to address the things that are within my control.
- My life has not been perfect, but I've learned many lessons and

have become stronger. With this growth, I'm ready to create the life I want to live.

- I have many strengths and qualities that make me lovable. I will start by loving myself.
- I won't always feel like this. These unpleasant feelings are information to create something different and better for myself.
- The more things I do to feel in control of my life, the better I will begin to feel.
- I'm going to be okay.

Or, once again, you can write your own specific new booster mantra—one that will help you create exactly the life you want. Take a few minutes to word it just the way you want it, and write it down.

Finally, take that new mantra and add some "because" statements to it. I'd like you to keep adding new ones as they occur to you, but take a few minutes to add at least three or four now:

I am going to be okay . . .

. . . because this time I'm going to do things differently and get the help I need.

. . . because I've felt this way in the past, and I got through it.

. . . because I'm willing to do whatever it takes to get me to the place I want to be.

. . . because I am loved, capable, and beautiful.

Now, as I've said already, I don't expect you to just jump on board with this new way of looking at the world and your life. It will take time for you to create the experiences that prove to you that your new mantra is true. I am going to help you with four exercises that can support your efforts to boost your brain chemistry.

Hindsight Is Twenty-Twenty

Remember the pitfall thought pattern called permanence? When you're gripped by any intense, unpleasant feeling, permanence is usually right there making it worse. Permanence says simply, "You're always going to feel like this!" and it's very hard not to believe it.

But it isn't true, and I'm going to help you prove it to yourself. Think back to a time when you felt really worried or angry about something that ended up being a short-lived problem. Maybe it was a nasty breakup that you thought you'd never get over. Or perhaps it was a fight with a friend, an argument at work, or a conflict with your family. Somehow or other, the matter eventually was resolved. Maybe you even thought, "What was I so worried about?" But when you were in it, the problem felt all-consuming. Impossibly heavy—and permanent.

Sit quietly for a minute and try to relive that painful time—including the memory of how nothing truly awful happened in the end. Allow yourself to absorb the truth: Those feelings were not permanent at all. Give yourself an image or a word that you associate with this lesson, and next time you're sure that you'll never feel any better than you do right now, picture the image or say the word. Don't let permanence sap your brain chemistry—use this exercise to fight back.

Talk to Your Heart

Imagine that your mind and your heart each have a voice and that they are having a conversation with each other. Your heart represents the way you feel, which sometimes includes pitfall thought patterns and unpleasant feelings. When you're hearing a voice telling you "It's always going to be this way" or "You can't possibly get through this," that's your heart talking. It might even be saying "Why bother?"

There's a reason the heart is giving us this message. Feelings are important information, and sometimes these despairing words are our way of telling ourselves: Make a change! This isn't working! Do something else!

So please don't ever ignore your heart. But do listen to what the mind is saying in response. When the emotional heart says, "I'm a terrible person and I hate myself," imagine the logical brain saying, "You're not terrible. You have good intentions in your life." When the heart says, "Why bother? Nothing will ever change," let the logical brain reply, "But we're embarking on a twenty-eight-day journey where we'll be doing things we're never done before. Imagine at least the possibility that we might feel different in ways we can't imagine now."

Let Your Feelings Float By

Imagine that you are sitting beside a peaceful river under a tree on a beautiful day. Feel yourself actually sitting there with the grass beneath you and your legs touching each other as you sit. Now, imagine that this river represents your mind and contains all of the thoughts and feelings you are experiencing at the present moment. Feel the separation between yourself and the river. What's floating by may be what you are thinking and feeling, but it is not *you*. You are here on the riverbank, not there in the water.

Notice the difference between this *essence* of you, and your thoughts and feelings. Just observe them, letting each thought or feeling flow by. Look, there goes *I'm not good enough!* There goes *Nothing will ever change!* There goes *You can't lose weight, so don't even try.* There goes *No one will ever love you,* and *You fail at everything,* and *What's the point?* You might recognize all those thoughts and feelings, but sitting here on the riverbank, can you see that they are not *you*? Don't argue, scold, or try to change them. Just watch them flow on by. . . .

Just Do Something

I've saved the simplest exercise for last: *Just do something.* On days when you feel yourself falling into every one of the seven pitfall thought patterns and your life feels completely out of control, just add activities that bring the booster attributes of pleasure and productivity into your day. Pick a task, no matter how small—putting a book away that's been lying on your coffee table, taking the garbage out, maybe even just taking a shower. Tell yourself to do it and let yourself accomplish it. Then pick some form of pleasure—a silly movie, a five-minute walk, a phone call with a friend—and do that. If you're not sure what to do, look at the list of booster activities on page 208 and 223 and pick one. Any one. Sometimes it's just the doing that matters.

My personal favorite thing to do on a really bad day is to go to the movies in a baseball cap, by myself, in the middle of the afternoon. If going to a funny movie helps at least 20 percent of my brain to stop worrying, I'll take it! If doing something simple such as going to the car wash helps me feel productive, I'll take that, too! Sometimes just a little step forward is all you need.

Restoring Balance, Regaining Control: Michaela's Story

Michaela was the kind of person to whom everybody turned in a crisis. As an emergency room nurse, she was used to handling high-tension situations, perhaps because she had grown up in a home with an alcoholic mother who was constantly creating crises for the rest of the family to solve. This early experience had accustomed Michaela to what I think of as the dopamine roller-coaster, a continual pattern of jolting to attention in order to cope with an emergency, followed by a massive letdown as the crisis passed . . . only to be followed, sooner or later, by yet another crisis.

As a child, Michaela medicated against the constant assault on her dopamine reserves by developing a taste for fatty meats, french fries, and rich cheeses. Her high-fat diet didn't lead to weight gain because she was also an athlete, but I believe she developed the beginnings of a food addiction at that time.

Later, in college, Michaela felt lonely away from her family, even though she was also glad to be on her own. At this point, she acquired a taste for the banana-nut and chocolate-chip muffins in her local coffee shop, where she'd go to study and hang out so she wouldn't have to sit in her room alone. She eventually made friends, found a boyfriend whom she later married, and felt as though her college years had been a success. Still, she had also created a potential addiction to sweet and fatty foods.

Michaela put on a little weight after her two children were born and she had less time to play sports and work out. But things didn't start to spin out of control until her mother got sick—really sick—with a heart condition that required an operation and then a series of hospital stays. Although Michaela lived in a different city and had a family of her own, she tried to handle her mother's care long-distance when she could and would fly in when she had to. Around the same time, one of her daughters started having trouble in school and the other one broke her leg in a gymnastics accident. The daughters' difficulties plus Michaela's absences naturally put a strain on Michaela's marriage and on the relationships at her job. By the time she came to me, Michaela felt that her life had spiraled completely out of control.

"I've gained fifty pounds in the past six months," Michaela confessed as she sat restlessly in my office chair. She was a study in contradiction—fidgety and agitated one moment, listless and exhausted the next. "I can't keep up with anything, my whole life's falling apart, I'm a total mess—and look how fat I am!" She started to cry, trying to gulp out an apology through her tears. "I'm sorry, Dr Mike, I don't know what to do, but I can't believe how badly I've screwed everything up. . . ."

Michaela was clearly struggling with multiple problems. She needed to figure out how to set boundaries with her mother, how to resolve things with her husband, and how to reconnect with her daughters, both of whom felt abandoned by what looked to them like their mother's preference for her own mother over them. She also needed to regain control of her relationship with food. It looked to me as though she had developed addictions to both high-fat and sweet, starchy foods in a desperate attempt to replenish the serotonin and dopamine that her high-stress, crisis-ridden life had depleted.

Michaela started the Diet Rehab program like anybody else: adding booster foods and activities without taking anything away. Because she was so depleted, I would have liked her to add as many boosters to her life and diet as possible, but I also saw that Michaela felt too over-whelmed even to do what my other patients had done. Suggesting a version of Cindy's nightly bath to her would have felt as out of the question as asking her to run a marathon. Mentioning Jim's hiking club would have been an insult, showing just how little I understood about how stressed, exhausted, and overwhelmed she felt. "You don't under-stand, Dr Mike," she kept saying. "I can't do *anything*. I could barely make it here!"

So we started small. We added just a five-minute walk to her after-noon or a cup of hot water with lemon when she felt like she couldn't take one more minute of work. And she agreed to try driving a new way home from work, which added a little dopamine-boosting newness while also helping her to avoid the fast-food restaurants that were ha-bitual and mindless traps. Of course, I made sure to reassure Michaela that she was not going to have to even consider giving up a single bite of muffin or a single order of french fries until she could do so without feeling the pain of withdrawal.

Michaela's road back to health was a long one, and it involved mak-ing a series of changes in her life, her mantra, and her relationships, as well as in her diet. But by day twenty-eight of Diet Rehab, without giv-ing up anything she wasn't ready to let go of, she had lost eight pounds and was beginning to feel less out of control. A double deficiency is a powerful challenge, but Michaela proved to be a powerful woman. By taking small steps at first, she got herself on the road to recovery. I was proud of her—but more important, she was proud of herself.

Feeding Your Brain to Control Your Life

It's a terrible feeling to be starving for everything. It's hard not to blame yourself for your predicament, even as you feel too depressed, insecure, and confused to take steps to change it. If you are starving for serotonin and desperate for dopamine, I feel for the discomfort you are in—but I want to assure you, there is a solution to your problem. Commit to the first day of the 28-day Diet Rehab program, and then, when that day is done, commit to the second day, and then the third, and then the fourth. Maybe it will be easier to make the commitment knowing that you don't have to give up *anything* until you're ready to do so. When the time is right, you'll take the next step—and regain control of your life.

PART III

Free Yourself From Food Addiction

7

Obsessive Eating: Seeking Security

When Jennifer first walked into my office, no one would have pegged her as an insecure woman whose mantra was *I'm not safe*. She was dressed beautifully in designer clothes and had a chic Beverly Hills haircut. Recently divorced, Jennifer was frustrated by the unsatisfying relationships she kept entering and by her ongoing tug-of-war with food.

Just as no one could have seen through to Jennifer's insecurities, no one would ever have suspected her addiction to food. Yet for Jennifer, each day was one long battle. At every meal, she fought to restrict her diet to the number of calories she had determined was appropriate for the weight she wanted to maintain. In the morning she struggled to keep from picking up snacks at the newsstand in her building's lobby. On her way home from work, she fought to prevent herself from stopping at the doughnut shop. Although Jennifer was slender and fit, she was anything but comfortable with food.

As I got to know Jennifer, I discovered that in middle school she had been mildly anorexic, followed by bouts of bulimia during high school and college. Now her anxieties took the form of constant diets and obsessive exercise. If she gained so much as a quarter pound, she began to panic. If she missed even a single day at the gym, she was sure that she was on her way to "looking fat and ugly." And if she ever did slip and violate her strict regime, she starved herself for days afterward, desperate to make up for what she saw as lost ground.

Jennifer's anxiety and her obsessive relationship to food were characteristic of someone who's short on serotonin. I encouraged her to consume more serotonin booster foods and tried to help her change her mantra. But the key for Jennifer was to tackle the addictive habits she developed. She needed to prove to herself that food was safe for her—indeed, that the world was safe.

As a cognitive-behavioral therapist I am fascinated by the interaction between behavior and attitudes. I know that the route to changing your thoughts and feelings is often to change the way you act. Actions can actually lead us to think differently—or they can reinforce the thoughts we already have.

Jennifer experienced the world as a frightening place and, consequently, she was continually anxious. She experienced food as a powerful force that could disrupt her body and her life, and as a result, she feared that, too. My agenda was to help her prove to herself that she could give up some of her obsessive behaviors and take steps toward changing her thinking without risking her safety.

Obsessive Eating and Serotonin

People who show obsessive eating behaviors usually also have a serotonin deficiency. So if you scored high on the serotonin-hungry quiz in Chapter 4, you may find that you're also trapped in obsessive behaviors. This can be one of many unique presentations of low serotonin. If you did not score high on the serotonin-hungry quiz in Chapter 4 and also do not score high on the obsessive eating quiz below, feel free to skip to Chapter 8.

Obsessive behaviors usually appear as an effort to regain a sense of control and safety through our actions. We're seeking security, predictability, and stability, hoping that if we control our food intake, we can control our lives.

The serotonin booster foods listed on page 204 in Chapter 12 will help reduce your anxiety, which should automatically help you let go of obsessive behaviors. You will also find some great serotonin booster meal and snack suggestions on page 243. In this chapter, I'll give you some additional support in overcoming food-related obsessions. Let's start by learning whether you *are* an obsessive eater. Take the following quiz to find out.

Am I an Obsessive Eater?

Take a look at the following list. Circle every item that applies to you.

1. I need to eat the exact same thing every day.
2. I feel extremely out of sorts, moody, or anxious when I can't get my usual choice of breakfast, lunch, or dinner.
3. I must sit and eat in the same spot every day.
4. I often turn down restaurant invitations because I prefer to eat a particular food at a particular time.
5. I have to have my own set of cutlery.
6. I can't eat certain colored foods.
7. I tell people I have an allergy when I've never been tested and there's no physical evidence I have one.
8. I don't like different foods to touch on my plate.
9. I have a way of eating that other people consider strange.
10. I weigh my food (and have not been told to do so by a professional).
11. I get very anxious if I can't complete my exercise routine every day.
12. I keep a calorie count in my head all the time.

13. If I eat something on my "forbidden" list, I starve myself for a while or double my exercise routine.
14. When I see someone in good shape, I have to find out what they eat.
15. I sometimes crave foods so badly I cry.
16. I don't allow myself to eat until I've showered/finished work/cleaned the house/done my rituals.
17. I like to go on juice or supplement-based fasts more than once a year.
18. I think the key to weight loss is eating no fat or carbs whatsoever.
19. I hide the evidence of my eating (packaging, dirty plates).
20. I prefer to cook for others and watch them eat rather than eat myself.
21. I often try to push food on my friends so I feel less guilty.
22. I bring my own food with me on occasions because I am fearful of new foods.
23. I have suffered from some form of anorexia or bulimia.
24. I have other non-food rituals I have to perform to feel safe.
25. I am extremely adamant about my foods being a certain brand or from a certain restaurant.

If you checked any of these, your eating behavior has some obsessive qualities, and the interventions outlined in this chapter will help you to gradually let them go. If your compulsive rituals take up a significant amount of time, if you find yourself unable to make even slight changes to them, or if your obsessions are extremely anxiety-provoking, consult a psychiatrist for screening and possible treatment of obsessive-compulsive disorder. If you are currently suffering from anorexia or bulimia, these are potentially life-threatening disorders that need immediate, professional treatment. See a mental health professional or go to my website—www.drmikedow.com—for treatment referrals.

How Do I Let Go?

The good news here is that, just as you gradually learned these obsessive rituals around food, you can also gradually unlearn them. If you
have gravitated toward obsessive patterns around food, then we look
at that as information indicating that you need more stability, predictability, or peace in your life. Luckily, the serotonin boosters listed on
pages 204 and 208 will help you to put the source of stability, predictability, or peace where it belongs: in your relationships, your sense of
purpose in your life, and confidence in yourself. These changes will
take place as you embark on your own Diet Rehab, and they will also
make the following obsessive-busting interventions more and more
achievable.

As you now know, the most effective way to create change is through
changing your experience. Even if you have specific food rules, such
as foods not touching each other, you already *logically* know that your
health would not be in jeopardy if you did not stick to this rule. But
emotionally, it still feels scary. The following interventions will gradually teach the emotional part of you that you are, indeed, going to be
okay, even if you take a more relaxed attitude toward food.

1. Stop weighing, measuring, and calorie-counting today.

For some people, weighing and measuring can be a great way to remain
aware of what they're eating. But if you tend to obsess about your food,
you will probably benefit from throwing out the scales and ditching the
tape measure, and you should definitely stop counting calories and
measuring food.

It may seem counterintuitive to let go of those methods of control,
but we're trying to switch from a world of restrictions to a universe
of abundance in which you can eat what you want and have what you
need. Take a leap of faith with me and begin to act as though you don't

need to weigh, measure, and count, because everything you want is simply going to work for you.

Set yourself up for success by starting small. Begin with a low-anxiety situation, such as a dinner where you are eating by yourself. Tell yourself, *just for this meal*, I will not count calories. After making yourself a reasonably sized, balanced meal, throw out the boxes with the nutritional information.

Throughout your meal, I want you to have a conversation with yourself in your head. Perhaps the emotional part of you says, "I'm feeling anxious. If I don't calculate the exact amount of calories, I'm not going to be okay." Then imagine the logical part of you replying, "That may be the way you're feeling right now, and this makes sense, as you've been engaging in this behavior for years. But logically, you know that there is actually nothing dangerous about not counting calories when this is a reasonable meal that has the nutritional elements you need. You're going to be okay."

Every time you do this, the emotional part of you will begin to become less anxious. Perhaps just a small amount will change, but you will be at least slightly less anxious than before. And the person teaching you this lesson is yourself, because your experience will begin to turn off that fear.

After you've mastered that first meal, do another. And then baby-step your way to gradually bigger steps, like not counting calories when you're eating with a group. If you're listening to how your body feels, and you know you're making healthy decisions about the foods you know your body needs, you'll be well on your way to managing your anxiety. The resulting lesson will be, "I am a resourceful and strong person. I'm working on this, and I'm teaching myself that I can handle what life throws at me." Allow this improvement in self-worth to help you achieve your goals in all areas of your life.

2. Change one thing about your food rituals or habits, just to prove to yourself that you can.

One of my patients learned the benefits of this involuntarily. Spencer was a successful forty-year-old lawyer who lived in a constant state of crippling anxiety. He was obsessed with the idea that he might screw up at work, or that if he left the office before ten p.m., he wasn't working hard enough. Spencer had always struggled with his weight and got up at five every morning to work out. But his eating rituals were so boring to his palate and so unsatisfying that he often craved fast food and wasted a lot of time and stress with this mental struggle. If he slipped up and ate something "off menu," he made himself run five miles. He told me that once he'd gone running at two a.m. because he'd eaten some fries.

Every night Spencer ordered in the exact same steak salad from the same place for dinner at his desk. Then one night disaster struck, as the restaurant changed the menu. Even though he begged and pleaded and finally became furious, the restaurant's new chef wouldn't make the old salad.

"I was so upset my palms were sweating!" Spencer told me. "I couldn't get any work done! I needed my salad to feel okay. It's hard to explain, but it was the only thing I ever wanted to eat for dinner. It was perfect and I always felt so good eating it."

Spencer had gotten used to calming himself with food. For him, eating was an island of order and security in his hectic, frenzied life. As a child, Spencer turned to sugar and carbs to help medicate a general feeling of unpredictability and chaos during his parents' divorce. Keeping rigid control over his eating helped him feel in command, but underneath the rationality he was trying to impose lurked an addiction to serotonin-releasing foods that Spencer desperately needed to help balance his brain chemistry.

First, I helped Spencer to see what emotions he was placing on that steak salad. "Knowing exactly what I'm getting" was really a sense of familiarity and stability. Spencer and I spent some time coming up with other places to put this emotional need, so we could take the need away from the food. Luckily, his serotonin boosters helped him to meet this need by calling friends, forgiving his parents, and taking a walk outside every day. These boosters all gave Spencer an overall feeling of "I'm going to be okay."

Meanwhile, Spencer had embarked upon a serious research project: calling around restaurants looking for a steak salad like his favorite. Sadly for him, he found that no one made it the way the old place did. He ended up ordering a steak with pepper sauce and grilled vegetables on the side.

We had rehearsed the way Spencer would get through this challenge of eating a new food. I instructed Spencer to have a conversation in his head between the logical and emotional sides of himself. So when the emotional side said, "I can't eat this. This is not the way it's supposed to be!" Spencer's logical side would reply, "I know this is hard, but you know that this new steak salad is not going to harm you. Every bite will be easier than the last and will help you to feel one percent less anxious."

In many ways, Spencer was being his own loving parent to his own inner, tantrum-throwing child. Although it wasn't easy, this exercise helped Spencer to get through the experience. In the end, he was surprised to discover how delicious the new dish was.

"When I was eating the new meal, I realized I was really paying attention to the flavors!" Spencer told me. "It's strange, I felt really happy and proud of myself afterward. I realized I would have felt weird if people had seen me eating the same salad every night. Of course no one ever did because I had this ritual of eating it alone at my desk. But now, trying something new, I felt free. I knew then maybe I could let go a little and it wouldn't kill me—I might even enjoy it. One night I even called my colleagues and we ate dinner together. I was still at work until ten p.m., but at least I'm taking baby steps!"

3. If rituals around food make you feel safe, create a new ritual that is not organized around food.

If you find yourself using repetitive behavior around food, transfer some of that energy to the relationships in your life. Having a ritualized date night with your significant other or a regular night out with your best friends works as a great replacement therapy.

Bethany, thirty-one, was obsessed with juice fasts. She seemed to be doing one every other week, or else an all-soup week to help "cleanse." What I could see was that rather than supporting her system, Bethany was starving herself.

When I asked Bethany to share her feelings about herself and what she ate, she shook her head miserably. "I'm fat," she said simply, referring to the ten to fifteen pounds she was constantly battling. "And if I eat like a regular person, I'll be huge! I know I will. I need to control my eating this way, or I'll blow up."

Actually, the truth was just the opposite: Bethany was ruining her metabolism with self-starvation, encouraging her body to cling to every ounce of fat she had and every measly calorie she consumed. On her no-carb diet, Bethany never had the energy to exercise, so her already-low serotonin levels weren't getting a boost there, either.

Despite Bethany's protests, I took a detour away from talking about food and weight and onto emotions and relationships. In the beginning, she didn't really see how they were all related. But I asked her, "What is it you really want, Bethany?"

Bethany told me how what she really wanted most of all was to be in a loving relationship with a man who loved her. And then I asked about how her obsessive juice fasts were helping her to manifest her most important goal. When Bethany told me that she needed to get these last ten or fifteen pounds off, I replied, "So your current mantra is: I'm fat and no one will love me like this." She smiled and acknowledged that I was spot on.

We then looked at how her self-critical mantra affected her achievement of long-term, long-lasting weight loss. Ironically, her mantra was making it harder, not easier, to lose weight. When we come from a place of judging ourselves and believing we're unlovable, that depletes our serotonin. And guess what we need to do when that serotonin goes down? We feel compelled to eat carbs and sugar, and we certainly don't feel like exercising.

To Bethany, losing ten to fifteen pounds was the precondition for being loved. In our work together, we discovered that it was actually the other way around: Feeling lovable was the precondition for losing ten to fifteen pounds. If serotonin boosters could help Bethany to *feel* loved, then she actually wouldn't need to go on juice fasts. And instead of just getting love through romantic relationships—which are largely outside of our control—we looked at the relationships that Bethany had more control over.

We examined how establishing a girls' takeout and TV night could actually help Bethany to not feel so alone. When she was with her girl-friends, they always gave her the sense that what she was going through wasn't all that unusual. We all struggle with self-worth from time to time. More important, Bethany realized how much love she already had in her life.

The other serotonin booster for Bethany was creating a Monday night yoga ritual. The calming and spiritual nature of the exercise was very healing for her, while the regularity and repetitiveness of the movements reassured Bethany and made her feel secure. Of course, it helped that yoga itself is a serotonin booster. For Bethany, it was the perfect activity, and best of all, she could practice it herself at home whenever she felt anxious. When she was tempted to self-medicate with carbs and candy, she could actually do something else that was good for her while satisfying the craving for a serotonin boost.

With this support and love, Bethany gave up her ritualistic juice fasts in favor of a sustainable way of eating. She had shifted from the sprint mentality to a marathon one. In the end, Bethany ended up losing about eight pounds and keeping it off for the long-term. It wasn't her "ideal" weight, but it definitely put her in the healthy category. And when Bethany was getting love from so many places in her life and realized she was worthy of love, she was perfectly happy with where she was.

Oh, and Bethany is now dating *and* eating solid foods every day. That's a win-win!

4. If you feel anxious at just the thought of not having total control of your diet, delegate responsibility to a friend who's willing to choose a new, healthy meal for you once a week.

Vivian was a forty-three-year-old marketing executive who struggled both with her weight and with obsessive thoughts about eating. Every day she liked to bring to work her own tuna salad, made her own particular way. She sometimes thought about eating something different or going out to lunch, but somehow she got stuck and felt antsy if she didn't stick to her routine.

I suggested to her that she literally give over control of her eating to a friend—just one meal per week—but even the thought of that upset her. Later she told me that it was as though the "private time" that she spent with her food rituals was being snatched away from her.

Vivian was tired of obsessing about her food choices, though, so she finally agreed to try this suggestion. "When I let my girlfriend decide what I would eat at lunch, I felt so angry!" she told me after her first attempt. "It was ridiculous! I'd actually *asked* her to do it, so I don't know what came over me, but I was mad."

With Vivian's overwhelming success in her work life, I wasn't surprised that giving up some personal control was a struggle for her. In some ways, it was admitting she had a weakness. But to Vivian, admitting that she was a human being who needed help every now and again was therapeutic in and of itself. In fact, Vivian's girlfriend said she felt relieved. She had always perceived Vivian as perfect and sometimes was a little afraid to confide in her. Now she felt able to get even closer to her.

After a few weeks, Vivian and her girlfriend called their Wednesday lunches "hump day lunch." The first two weeks were hard, but after that, it was quite easy. She had replaced her food ritual with a fun Wednesday lunch where she and her friend would try a new restaurant, celebrate their week, and plan for their weekends. This ended up being a much more effective serotonin booster that helped Vivian to create the life she actually wanted to live. After another month, they agreed to take turns picking new restaurants for their Wednesday outings, because going to new places and eating new things were no longer anxiety-provoking for Vivian. In fact, she looked forward to it. Ironically, the very ways she had been trying to make herself feel safe had only increased her anxiety. Opening up and becoming less isolated and more flexible paradoxically made Vivian feel safer.

Another benefit of changing her eating behaviors and improving her relationships was that Vivian felt more satisfied and therefore less likely to snack. She found she didn't need the calming sugar fixes that had kept her twenty pounds overweight since she was twenty-five. A couple of the other serotonin boosters, such as a five-minute meditation that she downloaded onto her iPod, were extra tools in her toolbox. In the end, Vivian not only gave up her obsessive ritual but also actually got what she was really needing in her life.

5. Shake up your food choices by flipping a coin. When it comes up heads, eat as you normally do. When it comes up tails, force yourself to make a new choice.

This works for excessive exercise plans and obsessive calorie-counting, too. For example, if you usually run five miles or hit the gym for an hour daily, take a day off when the coin lands on tails. Or work up to the day off with baby steps, such as limiting yourself to a brisk walk instead of your demanding routine.

All of these behavior-changing exercises can achieve two goals. First, you'll learn that even if you don't have total control over your food, you'll be all right. Second, you'll be forced to focus your control issues less on food and more on other sources of stability and pleasure: family, home life, work, and your own happiness.

Set Yourself Up for Success

Remember, the first time you do something will always be harder than the second, or third, or fourth time. As I said earlier, listen to your heart saying, "I can't do this!" while your logical mind says, "I'm just changing my routine, it won't hurt me." You can choose which voice to listen to, even though at first, your heart will be speaking much, much louder. But every time you listen to the logical voice, it gets one percent stronger.

Of course, the whole process is slow, because your emotional voice has ruled your eating for your whole life up until now. So be patient with yourself. Set yourself up to win this fight by being kind and compassionate with your emotions. They'll come around in the end!

8

Emotional Eating:
The Search for Joy

Dede was only seven pounds over her ideal weight, but those seven pounds took up virtually all of her attention. If Jenny's serotonin-deprived behavior in Chapter 7 was obsessive eating, Dede's dopamine- and serotonin-fueled pitfall was emotional eating. While Jenny was a prisoner of her fears, Dede was a slave to her beliefs that she was neither attractive nor lovable. "I'm not worth anything," her mantra declared—and Dede's hangdog look, her loose-fitting clothes, and her slumped shoulders shouted that message loud and clear.

As an emotional eater, Dede went for her serotonin and dopamine pitfall foods whenever she found confirmation of her negative self-concept. Of course, since she was constantly looking for that confirmation, she usually found it! Dede was so sure she was worthless that she confirmed that opinion for herself before the world could do it for her. If she met a man she might have been interested in, rather than flirt with him or pursue a relationship, she ate. If she had an opportunity for a promotion or a new job, rather than pursue the possibility, she ate.

If she spent a difficult Sunday with her mother, rather than either confront her mom or find a more satisfying way to spend her weekend, she ate.

Dede exercised excessively, so she was only seven pounds past her ideal weight. Yet her relationship with food was no less addictive than that of my more severely overweight patients. In many ways, food dominated Dede's life even more than it did some of theirs.

As with Jenny, my goal with Dede was to give her situations in which she could prove to herself that her pitfall mantra was incorrect and that her core beliefs were wrong. If Dede could truly grasp the possibility that she was lovable and worthy, she would be well on her way to freeing herself from the addictive triggers that left her looking for solace in a bag of crisps.

One day, the guy Dede had liked for a long time but always avoided started dating a new woman. Dede responded by eating a whole large pizza by herself. I asked her to go back and recount the moment she knew she wanted to eat. Simply the act of recognizing her trigger was helpful in getting Dede to see herself and her behavior with a new clarity. I also wanted Dede to rewrite her story, asking "What would the ideal Dede with a booster mantra have done in that moment?"

I had Dede practice writing down all the things she felt good about in her life. Every day I asked her to add something to the list. She began reluctantly with "My job is okay," but by day ten she was writing about her love of fashion and how happy she was to have her best girlfriend in her life.

During the third week, Dede's mom spent all afternoon with Dede complaining about her problems. In the past Dede would have left her mom's house feeling both drained and somehow guilty for her very existence. Normally by the time she neared home, she'd know she needed ice cream and she'd stop at the store for a pint of chocolate-chip and a can of whipped cream for topping. But this time, Dede gave her mom a few minutes of encouragement and compassionate listening, but not so much that Dede felt drained. Then she got up and said it was time she got home. As she walked to her car, she felt a little guilty. But she felt okay—not great, but fine—and she didn't need the ice cream.

The following week, when Dede's mom started in on her complaining, she also criticized Dede for not listening to her problems. But this time Dede had a new answer for her mom.

"I love you, mom," she said. "But I think we both need to have some fun together. Sometimes I just feel so overwhelmed at the end of a long work day. It has nothing to do with not *wanting* to listen. It's just that sometimes, I *can't*." Dede even told her mother about the concept of "paralysis-analysis," where you keep ruminating about your problems without ever really moving on.

Dede then pulled a DVD out of her bag—a funny romantic comedy with an actor they both liked—and suggested that they sit down together to watch it. Her mom was surprisingly upbeat afterward, and Dede knew she'd taken a big step toward letting go of emotional eating.

Doing something that gives you a sense of pleasure like watching a movie can be a simple yet effective strategy for eating more responsibly. Dede had also tested her ability to leave herself out of her mom's paralysis-analysis pitfall style of thinking, and she had discovered that nothing awful had happened.

Six weeks later, Dede told me she'd met a man. There was a new guy working in her building. Dede thought he was cute, but she never thought he'd be attracted to her. She hadn't felt comfortable being flirtatious, but she had managed to look him in the eye and smile.

Dede continued to work on standing up for herself, feeling like a worthwhile person and not suppressing her emotions while she ate her booster foods and did the booster activities I'd recommended in her Diet Rehab plan. She started every morning with twenty minutes of learning French with an online program and opened a savings account for her dream trip to Paris. Dede needed these booster activities to remind herself that her life was full of experiences to look forward to—experiences that she could choose to create. When she chose to cook booster foods at home instead of medicating her feelings with expensive takeout, she put the five dollars she had saved into her Paris fund. She wasn't focusing on what she was taking away but on what she was choosing to add.

As she reprogrammed her behavior, Dede began to notice she didn't feel those urges to automatically eat whenever she experienced a nasty moment or a low feeling. In fact, she felt those lows less and less often. She became friendly with the man in her office, and he asked her out for a drink.

One day she noticed four of the extra seven pounds she had carried around for years were gone. And they stayed gone. But most important, Dede's state of mind was improved. She even liked herself enough to realize the remaining three pounds were not noticeable or worth thinking about. Her emotional eating habit was broken and she was able to let go and enjoy herself.

Am I an Emotional Eater?

Sometimes I think that we've all been trained to eat in response to emotions. Commercials show people smiling and having a great time after they've eaten some sugary doughnuts, a packaged bag of crisps, or a can of soda. We're even taught to associate life's happiest moments—such as the cake on your birthday—with food.

Of course, there's nothing wrong with occasionally celebrating or comforting yourself with food. But I want your choices to be conscious and deliberate ones. Some treats, like the occasional piece of birthday cake, can continue to be celebratory parts of your life. But if you need something to make you feel better every day, then I want you to look to a serotonin or dopamine booster food, or better yet, an activity. A concrete action will help you tackle the root cause of your emotional eating by getting the peace or excitement you're really hungry for.

Some of the strategies at the end of this chapter—whether you're low on serotonin, dopamine, or both—are especially helpful if you struggle with emotional eating. But let's start by finding out whether emotional eating is an issue in your life. Take the following quiz to find out.

Am I an Emotional Eater? A Quiz

Take a look at the following list. Circle every item that applies to you.

1. I have always felt guilty about eating.
2. When I was little, I ate more than the other kids.
3. I have at least one friend who makes me feel bad, but I can't seem to let him or her go.
4. I had a difficult relationship with my family.
5. I'm often lonely.
6. When I eat, I'm not truly satisfied, even when I eat a lot.
7. I eat just to have something to do.
8. I always like to eat something when I get home, because it's comforting.
9. I eat when other people eat, even if I'm not hungry.
10. I feel powerless around food.
11. I often feel very down on myself.
12. I get very upset when I can't eat my favorite food.
13. My parents often rewarded me with food when I was a child.
14. I feel quite disconnected from my body sometimes.
15. I berate myself in front of the mirror a lot.
16. My desire to eat comes from above-the-neck emotional hunger, rather than below-the-neck physical hunger.
17. I have gone through phases of trying to limit my eating, but sometimes I eat a very large amount of food without really noticing.
18. I often eat in front of the TV.
19. I've noticed I'll crave my favorite pitfall foods when something unpleasant has happened.

20. I want to eat at weird times of the day and sometimes wake in the night, wanting to snack.
21. I sometimes feel overwhelmingly sad before eating.
22. Other people push me around and I always treat myself with food afterward.
23. I find it almost impossible to stand up for myself and I eat to cover how that makes me feel.
24. When I say no, I feel guilty—and I often eat to comfort myself.
25. I eat almost no calories during the day but then consume a lot at night.

If you checked one or more of the above questions, you have some form of emotional eating behavior, which probably indicates either low serotonin, low dopamine, or, in many cases, both. The interventions outlined in this chapter will help you to gradually let them go. Don't despair—you can break the cycle and change not only the way you feel about yourself but also the way you react to difficult, unpleasant, or overwhelming feelings. If you are unable to make even slight changes or experience any major symptoms of depression or anxiety, see a mental health professional or go to my website—www.drmikedow.com—for treatment referrals.

Emotional Eating and Your Brain Chemistry

If you're dopamine-deprived, you tend to feel as though life has lost its luster. You might feel empty and down or overwhelmed and drained. You might crave drama and thrills to lift you out of your slump, or you might just long for something pleasurable and fun to relieve the daily stress.

If you're serotonin-starved, you might feel anxious and on edge, worried about your work, relationships, or personal life simply slipping out of control. Or you might lack confidence and feel pessimistic, fearful that nothing will work out for you, or perhaps even certain that it won't.

If you're short on both types of brain chemicals, you may simply feel that life has gotten away from you. You might believe that you don't have the energy or clarity to make changes or pursue your goals—that it's all you can do just to get through the day.

In all of these cases, you may well engage in what I call emotional eating: eating in response not to physical hunger or nutritional need, but rather as the result of emotional challenges. Of course, as we have seen, emotional challenges are physical, too. When you feel depressed, overwhelmed, stressed, sad, blocked, or disregarded, your brain chemistry responds accordingly. Your stores of dopamine and serotonin are depleted, and you need more biochemical support for the challenges you're facing, making your desire to eat sweet, starchy, or fatty foods as much a physical response as the hunger your feel after hours of heavy physical labor.

The solution, as we have seen throughout this book, is to feed your brain with the foods and activities it needs to manufacture a nice, steady supply of the serotonin and dopamine on which it relies. Then you'll always feel "fed" and full, and you won't need quick fixes. Meanwhile, I can offer you some specific suggestions for rewriting your emotional eating patterns into healthier and more satisfying rhythms.

How Do I Start Feeling Full?

Luckily, if you load your life with the serotonin and dopamine booster foods and activities I suggest in Chapters 12 and 13, a lot of your emotional eating will disappear on its own. Your brain chemicals will be replenished in a healthy, stable way, and you simply won't feel the pull of emotional eating as you did before.

The other way to start feeling full is to focus on specific actions that will make you feel positive and satisfied about your life. Since the most effective way to create change is through changing your experience, anything you do to improve your life will alter the way you feel about food. The more important other experiences become, the less important eating will seem—and that process will happen naturally, and without effort. If you'd like to let go of some of your emotional eating patterns, give one of the following suggestions a try.

1. YOU ARE GOOD ENOUGH

Do one thing that will make you feel "good enough" today. You might push yourself to just smile or say hello to someone in the elevator, make a five-dollar donation to an animal rescue group or pediatric cancer foundation, or call a friend who always seems to "get you." Now you feel a sense of peace, which you'll remember was one of the seven booster attributes I listed on page 63. Connecting to your ability to make a difference reminds you how many worthy and lovable qualities you have. There's also nothing wrong with trying to make yourself feel as good as possible on the outside when you feel lousy on the inside. When I feel down or have been mourning a breakup, those are some of the moments when I decide to put on my favorite shirt, shave, and comb my hair. And there's a little of that other booster attribute: pride.

2. SIGN UP FOR YOUR FUTURE

Take a positive step toward a goal by trying something new. If you've always wanted to learn to paint, sign up for classes. If you've secretly always yearned to be a dancer but thought you weren't graceful enough, find a beginner's class and enroll today. If you have a dream vacation, open a savings account. Notice how you're filling your life with two more of the seven booster attributes: productivity and purpose. You can find more suggestions for booster activities in Chapters 12 and 13.

3. DETACH FROM SITUATIONS THAT DRAIN YOU

In my experience, people who are prone to emotional eating are often the caretakers in a relationship. If that sounds like you, try this: Next time you're with people who are talking about their problems, see what happens if you don't do anything. Try to tolerate their unhappiness without trying to fix it. This should also help you build tolerance against your own moods next time you feel unhappy, and so your unhappiness will be less likely to translate into hunger. You don't have to fix anything. You also have the right to surround yourself with people who nourish you and fill your life with two of the seven booster attributes: power and peace.

4. INVITE AND WRITE SOME LOVE LETTERS

Ask the five people closest to you in the world to e-mail you the three things they like best about you. Notice your reactions when you read the e-mails. Do you feel like arguing with them? Pointing out your flaws? Wondering why they picked those good qualities and not others of which you are prouder or that you wish you had? Take some time to notice how many of your thoughts had to do with fears of people mocking you or dismissing you rather than expressing their appreciation. Then write back at least a brief love note to each participant, expressing your gratitude for the joy they bring into your life.

5. MEDITATE

Engage in mindful meditation, where you practice simply observing your feelings rather than trying to respond to them. Take five minutes a day to just sit quietly and practice watching your thoughts come and go. You can build up to thirty minutes or longer with practice, but start slowly, as sometimes it can be tough to quiet your thoughts. Some people find it helpful to choose a word or phrase they enjoy and repeat it in time with their deep breathing. You can go to drmikedow.com to download a guided meditation. I always tell my patients, "If you don't take your feelings so personally, your feelings won't take you so personally!" That extra distance from your feelings might give you a little more space to start making other decisions around food. You'll let go of the pitfall of paralysis-analysis while increasing peace, one of the booster attributes.

6. TAKE A MINDFUL WALK

Grab the dog, call a friend, or simply plug in your iPod and take a brisk walk around the block *before* you give in to your emotional eating urge. As you walk, really feel your body. Feel your legs move and notice the tingle in your feet as they hit the road. Feel your breathing and notice how the air smells. Listen to the sound of the birds or passing cars. Pay attention to the way the light hits the trees. Say hello to anyone you pass, smiling and looking them in the eye. Pick up your feet, don't shuffle, and, if you can, adjust your posture so you're standing tall as you walk. Move as though you feel good about yourself, even if you don't. Studies show that with practice, behaving as though you feel good actually *makes* you feel good. You've lifted your mood with the booster attributes of power, pride, and pleasure, which might replenish your brain chemistry instead of the food you would normally choose.

7. DISTRACT YOURSELF

Most cravings last about two minutes and are satisfied by about four bites. So if you can just distract yourself for a little while, you might simply forget about being hungry. Try the booster activities on pages 208 and 224, or do one of the items on the following list:

Brush your teeth
Clean your kitchen counters
Chew some sugar-free gum
Floss
Go online and read a blog post
Listen to an uplifting song, and if you can, dance to it
Plan a family day out
Put on a teeth-whitening strip
Take a shower
Unload the dishwasher
Write a quick friendly e-mail to someone you like

8. MAKE A GRATITUDE LIST

Sit down and write a list beginning with the words, "I am grateful because . . ." and then think about everything that is good in your life, no matter how small. It could be anything from "I have nice hair" to "I have a great relationship with my son" to "The weather was good today." As soon as you start looking for things to feel good about, you'll be surprised how many there are. Keep the list with you and add to it whenever you feel moved to do so. Read it whenever you feel like emotionally eating and see if you can feel even a little bit of serotonin or dopamine flooding back into your brain.

9. GIVE YOURSELF A BREAK

We often think that the best way to move forward is to criticize ourselves for anything we do wrong, hoping to keep ourselves in line and avoid the same mistakes in the future. In fact, the best way to improve is exactly the opposite: to forgive ourselves for our mistakes and let them go as quickly as possible, and to focus on what we've done right. Several studies in sports psychology have found that if an athlete makes a mistake, self-talk such as "I'm trying so hard!" and "I don't give up, good for me!" is far more useful than "I just dropped the ball—what an idiot," or "I shouldn't have done that."

I suggest the same approach to you: Whatever your results with regard to emotional eating, focus on what you've done right, even if it seems like merely a tiny piece of the big picture. Self-criticism only lowers your serotonin levels, leaving you feeling low and then making you want to emotionally eat again.

10. BE MINDFUL

One of the greatest gifts we can give ourselves—in the midst of any grief, fear, anxiety, or depression—is to just be here now. The present moment is the only place where we can really be fully at peace, the place where everything just *is*, and we don't have to imagine what might be or will be, where we don't have to fret about what we've just done or failed to do. In the present, we just *are*. If you can be mindful and eat mindfully—really tasting and savoring your food—you can indulge in the pleasure of the food so that even if eating is an emotional choice, you can satisfy the craving in a few bites rather than continuing past the point where you don't feel any pleasure in it.

Here's an exercise in mindfulness that might give you some practice in mindful eating:

Take a raisin, grape, or similar small food, such as a fruit or nut, and put it on your tongue. Sit quietly with your eyes closed and do not chew. Simply let the food sit in your mouth. Notice any flavors or smells. Really experience the grape's smooth, elastic skin or the leathery tough surface of the raisin. Feel the food's texture on your tongue. Roll it around in your mouth and taste the flavors as it warms up. Keeping your eyes closed, really notice the changes in texture and flavor as you slowly start to chew. Chew the food at least fifty times—more, if you can—to notice how it feels to keep food in your mouth rather than swallowing it instantly. When you do swallow, feel the food travel down your throat and enter your stomach. Sit quietly for a moment to absorb the sensations fully. You can also download a guided mindful eating track from www.drmikedow.com.

Putting Your Emotions in Perspective

As a therapist, I want my patients to get in touch with their feelings—to celebrate and honor their emotions. But I also want them to keep their feelings in perspective, rather than letting them run their lives.

I want the same thing for you. I want you to respect your feelings, but I want you also to listen to your rational side, the one that helps you have a different dialogue within your mind and heart. If you give yourself the booster attributes, foods, and activities that feed your brain chemistry and nourish your life, your feelings will get the support they need, and you'll be able to let go of emotional eating almost without trying. Both your weight and your emotions will benefit.

9

Binge Eating: Regaining Control

When I met my patient Jenna at age twenty-eight, she was in tough shape. With circles under her eyes and the habit of constantly picking at her fingernails, she was clearly so anxious and in so much emotional pain she was barely functioning.

"I've always taken things very personally," she admitted. Jenna had a great memory and felt everything deeply. Every experience was almost painfully intense for her.

Jenna had come to me following a bad breakup. Unable to move on from the feelings of rejection, she had slipped back into her teenage habit of binge eating and now, locked in a cycle of strict diets and all-out gorging sessions, she had a hard time keeping self-hatred at bay.

Binge eaters may be either serotonin deficient or dopamine deprived, but most of the time they are both. Most binges are made up of both serotonin-releasing carbs and sugar plus dopamine-releasing fat, as evidenced by Jenna's binges of pizza, ice cream, candy, crackers, french fries, and soda.

The key to putting an end to compulsive eating is to create a feeling of abundance (no food is forbidden) and a sense of order (eating comes at regularly scheduled times, hungry or not). If you're a binge eater, you are by definition in the grip of intense spikes and crashes of various brain chemicals, as well as blood sugar, and you've long ago lost touch with genuine hunger. You might also feel a great deal of shame about your out-of-control eating. Encouraging you to eat three meals and two to three snacks every day—each and every day—is the first step in helping you regain control.

Jenna began her 28-day Diet Rehab plan with both serotonin and dopamine booster foods and activities, and with my encouragement for her to plan out most of her meals and snacks in advance. That way, she could feel more control over her eating and was less likely to slip into a binge.

But the first time Jenna came to see me after beginning Diet Rehab, she was sobbing.

"I was sure I'd get fat if I ate normally," she told me. "So I cut out the two snacks and skipped breakfast. Then I just felt like I couldn't do it anymore, so I ate."

"And what did you eat?" I asked.

"Bread. A whole loaf," she cried. "Then I punished myself for the next twelve hours by not eating anything, and that led to an even worse binge! I'll always be like this. It's just the way I'm made! I'm weak and oversensitive. Why can't I just get over things like other people? Why don't I have any self-control?"

Gently I explained to her that her problem was not her sensitivity. Rather, it was that she hadn't learned to celebrate and be proud of who she really was. Instead, she constantly berated herself, bringing her mood down lower than ever. What she needed was a steady stream of serotonin and dopamine boosters and some cognitive-behavioral tools to help her make the decisions she truly chose and then to stick to them.

"You are not allowed to feel bad about relapsing," I told her firmly. "And I also don't want you skipping any meals or snacks, whether you binge or not. If you relapse again, you will. If you relapse twenty times, you will. One day you won't. And meanwhile, you'll keep eating normally. Now move on to planning tonight's snack and meal. Tomorrow is another day, and you can take this a day at a time."

Together we worked on changing Jenna's low opinion of herself. I had her meditating every morning for five to ten minutes as she practiced clearing her mind of thoughts and just observing her feelings as if from a distance. (Go to www.drmikedow.com for your own guided meditation session.) She also worked on changing her mantra of "I'm not good enough" to "I'm worth it." (For more on mantras, go to pages 84 and 118.)

To help reset Jenna's binge eating, I also made sure she kept a journal about her feelings along with everything she ate. I also made her throw out her scales and allowed her to weigh herself only once each week, in my office. We agreed to do blind weighing so that I alone would know her weight until twenty-eight days had passed. That's because Jenna was so obsessed about her weight that knowing it even weekly made her more anxious. Also, sometimes a person who has been starving and bingeing may see his or her weight go up before it goes down. I didn't want Jenna to feel discouraged.

And indeed, Jenna gained two pounds at first, simply from her body's reaction to regular eating. On a constant yo-yo of starving and bingeing, her metabolism had become sluggish, and she wasn't burning calories efficiently. But with support from the friends and family I encouraged her to confide in, Jenna didn't lapse back into her binge-starve cycle.

During this period I also helped Jenna learn to eat in public without panicking. Her fear of food and her tendency to binge in secret had made eating in restaurants and in front of people a difficult experience. First she went to a cozy little café for lunch. She had a Niçoise salad with dopamine-boosting tuna fish and egg slices and some serotonin-boosting chamomile tea. She took a book with her to help her feel less self-conscious about sitting alone.

The next time, she went to the café with a friend who knew all about her issues. Jenna felt anxious at first and even told me later that having her friend there had made her feel as though she should eat only half of her meal. She stuck to the plan and left the restaurant satisfied—but half an hour later, she wrote in her journal that she wanted to eat a whole chocolate cake. She had learned from keeping her food and mood journal in Diet Rehab that eating in public was one of her worst triggers. But then she looked at her meal plan and knew she could have a snack in two hours' time. Jenna relaxed and the chocolate cake remained on the store shelf.

After three weeks her body was stabilizing. She felt hungry at mealtimes and was then hugely relieved to find she was allowed to just eat a meal without guilt. Later in the evenings she felt that she didn't need to binge. She was satisfied. Leaving the daily guilt cycle behind, she began to feel better about herself and she saw herself as less isolated and more like other "normal" people.

By now, Jenna could eat in a restaurant without panicking. In fact, she went to a work lunch and instead of avoiding food in front of her intimidating clients and then gorging on fries afterward, she ate a healthy lunch and stuck to her plan.

Of course the triggers were still in Jenna's life. Her ex-boyfriend still haunted her. To Jenna, the way her relationship had ended confirmed the fear that she wasn't good enough. But now, with the self-esteem-boosting work she had done, Jenna saw that she had options. She could go on a dinner date and she could let a man fully into her life. She no longer had anything to hide. Knowing that she was no longer trapped in her secret binge-eating behavior gave Jenna the freedom to enjoy herself, while eating regular healthy meals reset Jenna's behavior and boosted her brain chemistry. Her increased serotonin and dopamine levels ensured that her mood stayed on an even keel.

Jenna lost five pounds over her twenty-eight days of Diet Rehab and has been slowly and steadily losing the next fifteen pounds toward her goal weight of 145 pounds. What was most surprising to Jenna was that she actually lost weight over the course of twenty-eight days, even though she was not allowed to skip any meals or even so much as a snack! Jenna had spent most of her life starving herself for half the week or more. It seemed ironic to her that by eating normally, she actually *lost* weight. But this is exactly what happens.

Why Am I Like This?

Binge eaters generally experience the world as a very intense place. They are often creative, deeply sensitive, intuitive types who are likely to have strong emotional reactions. These individuals often feel "different" or isolated due to their sensitivity and are prone to low feelings as a result. They might self-medicate with drugs, alcohol, or food, or simply isolate themselves from situations that they fear will provoke bad feelings. That's partly because someone who tries to self-medicate with a substance has never fully learned how to self-soothe. Where someone else might say, "You can handle this" or "You're better than that," the low-serotonin-and-dopamine binge eater doesn't have the brain chemical support or the childhood training to get through a challenging experience without a self-medicating binge.

Of course, the sensitivity that leads to these intense feelings also leads to artistic, political, and spiritual insight. Great artists, poets, musicians, and writers all share this trait, as do many spiritual leaders and humanitarians. Managing the low points of this sensitivity is important, however, and part of that is seeking a supportive plan that works for you. Diet Rehab, with its support for your brain chemistry and its booster activities, can help you find both the chemical and personal support you need.

The serotonin and dopamine booster foods listed on page 204 in Chapter 12 and on page 219 in Chapter 13 will help replenish your brain chemistry, which should ease the need to binge. In this chapter,

I'll also provide you with a range of approaches that can assist you in making calmer and less impulsive choices. The first step is to find out what role bingeing has in your eating habits. Take the following quiz to find out.

Am I a Binge Eater?

Take a look at the following list. Circle every item that applies to you.

1. I feel guilty, depressed, or ashamed after eating.
2. I eat to the point of feeling uncomfortably full or even of being in pain.
3. I eat what most people would consider a very large amount of food in a short amount of time.
4. I eat a large amount of food when I'm not physically hungry.
5. I avoid social situations where food is present.
6. When I eat, I'm often not truly satisfied, even when I eat a lot.
7. I attribute nearly all my success or failure to my weight.
8. I feel powerless around food.
9. I quite often feel very down on myself.
10. I feel a lack of control when I begin eating.
11. I enter a trancelike state when I begin eating.
12. I feel quite disconnected from my body sometimes.
13. I berate myself in front of the mirror a lot.
14. After a binge, I will compensate by restricting the amount of food I will eat the next meal or next day.
15. I often eat in front of the TV.
16. I eat very rapidly.
17. I've noticed I'll crave my favorite pitfall foods when something unpleasant has happened.
18. Most of my eating occurs late at night.
19. I eat very little food during the day.

20. I sometimes feel overwhelmingly sad before eating.
21. My binges occur in private because I'm embarrassed about how much I eat.
22. I have ritual foods that I will obtain to binge on.
23. I feel anxious once I begin thinking about obtaining my foods and my upcoming binge, but I feel that I can't do anything to stop it.
24. I pretend that the food I buy is not all for me in some way, such as going to different drive-through restaurants or telling the takeout people that I'll need more than one set of utensils.
25. I hoard foods—especially high-calorie, high-fat pitfall foods.

If you checked any of these, you may have difficulty with binge eating, which probably indicates either low serotonin, low dopamine, or, in many cases, both. The interventions outlined in this chapter will help you to gradually let go of these difficulties. If your binge eating is excessive, and if you find yourself unable to make even slight changes, consult a mental health professional for screening and treatment of binge-eating disorder. If you are currently suffering from anorexia or bulimia, be aware that these are potentially life-threatening disorders that need immediate, professional treatment. See a mental health professional or go to my website—www.drmikedow.com—for treatment referrals.

Ride the Wave

Think of your hunger as an overpowering wave that you want to learn to ride. When you introduce regular, planned eating, it's as though you're learning to surf and learning how to paddle. When you skip meals, it's as though you're helplessly hanging out on your board in the ocean. When the wave comes, you're not paddling, so it knocks you off your board and you're swept into the proverbial undertow of binge eating.

By contrast, people who eat regular meals are always paddling, so when their waves come, they surf them. Their waves are manageable, while for you, skipping meals leaves you open to drowning.

That's why I don't want you to think of yourself as "on a diet" or to allow yourself to feel deprived in any way. You'll be vulnerable to binges and will let the wave ride you instead of you riding it.

What's Your Trigger?

In a study on binge eating, researchers discovered twelve main triggers:

Tension—91 percent
Eating something—84 percent
Being alone—78 percent
Craving specific foods—78 percent
Thinking about food—75 percent
Going home—72 percent
Feeling bored and lonely—59 percent
Feeling hungry—44 percent
Drinking alcohol—44 percent
Going out with someone who might be a romantic partner—
    25 percent
Going to a party—22 percent

Think about your own triggers and write them down. It's important to be mindful of when you're most vulnerable, and it will also allow you to combat your triggers with booster activities. When you fill your life with things that promote healthy relationships while decreasing isolation and loneliness, you'll find that your triggers won't be as power-

DIET REHAB

ful. And, of course, booster foods eaten at regularly scheduled meals and snack times will help you to no longer be a prisoner to food and bingeing.

> ## Compulsive Eaters Come in All Shapes and Sizes
>
> Weight and binge eating are not really related. Most binge eaters are not overweight, and most obese people—some 90 to 95 percent—don't binge.

Be Kind to Yourself

If you binge, you may also have trouble asserting yourself. You might feel that you are never good enough. You may have standards that are quite high, and that you believe you do not meet. And you might isolate yourself from people or situations in which you would find yourself feeling as though you had fallen short or even failed.

That's why I'd like you to be as kind as possible to yourself, adding booster activities and foods and giving yourself all the support you can manage. Treat your state of mind as you would an innocent child. Recognize that your impulses are triggered by feeling low and, when you're mean to yourself, you feel lower.

I also want to encourage you to set achievable goals. Don't focus on the big picture of what you'd someday like to do. Pick something to accomplish this week. This is important both for weight-loss goals and for other tasks. Small, steady, measurable gains will make you feel better about yourself, your life, and your ability to succeed. Set yourself up for success by choosing this approach.

Breaking the Cycle of Fear and Fat

Often, if you binge, you're actually scared of food, because you think that the food itself will cause you to binge. You find yourself feeling paralyzed, thinking of food at every turn, terrified of the feelings that you might experience just from being around food.

The solution? An approach known as graded exposure therapy. With this method, you can go at your own pace and take very small steps toward freedom. I used this approach with Jenna when I had her eat out alone, then with a friend. Try the following exercise yourself to see how this technique might be helpful to you.

EXERCISE: FACE YOUR FEAR

1. Eat in front of someone at home (preferably this person is supportive and aware of your struggle).
2. Eat at a restaurant or café that you find comfortable and unintimidating with a good friend you feel you can trust and be relaxed with.
3. Go to the same place (or another you are equally comfortable with) and eat with people you're unsure of or who give you anxiety, such as a colleague or family member.
4. Choose a new restaurant and eat with a person or group that makes you anxious or tense, such as friends of friends you experience as intimidating, colleagues, or a difficult family member.

Repeat these steps until you can do each one without terrible anxiety. If a binge is triggered, accept that as part of the process, and go through the steps again without skipping the next meal or snack. Your goal is to feel somewhat less anxious and somewhat less frantic to escape. Moving away from avoidance one baby step at a time will help you to conquer your fear without being overwhelmed. Give yourself credit for any effort you make and for even the smallest improvement.

Rules to Live by for Binge Eaters

1. **Have a plan.** Binge eaters need to stick to a plan of three meals and two to three snacks every day. When filling out your food journal (see page 263), know that only the third snack of the day is optional for you. Map out what you will eat the next day and shop or plan for this in advance. I advise investing in lunch bags or boxes to take your food to work. Think ahead. If you're unprepared, you're more likely to fall into a binge.

2. **Never skip meals.** Punishing yourself by skipping a meal is the cornerstone of binge eating. You're setting yourself up this way. First come the low feelings of guilt, then the self-punishment and even lower feelings, then finally the real hunger hits you and you start to crave a binge.

3. **Enjoy food.** You don't have to eat food that's bland or unenjoyable. Remember, you are not allowed to beat yourself up or feel deprived on this plan. Find booster foods that you'll enjoy. When planning your meals, think about the flavors you really like. You can even find some great simple recipes on page 297 so you can create an entire meal out of boosters. You can even boost your brain chemistry with pancakes!

4. **Never say never.** If you say, "I'm never going to eat this food," it increases the possibility of a binge. Don't encourage impulse eating by keeping your trigger foods at home, but at the same time, never say "never" to them or they'll be calling your name from the store. Tell yourself, "I can have that later," or work a small amount of something you crave into tomorrow's meal plan.

5. **Keep a journal.** Writing down what you eat helps keep you accountable to yourself and whomever you choose to share your Diet Rehab journey with. Journaling is a key part of this program, so go to the journal section on page 263 and make sure you are keeping a full and honest track of your food.

6. **Weigh yourself only once a week.** Obsessing over the scale will expose you to emotional ups and downs that can trigger a binge. Everyone's weight varies a little throughout the day, so don't pay too much attention to each weekly weight reading. It's better to consider your weight over a period of four weeks or, better yet, a year.

7. **Find a friend.** One of the most common characteristics of binge eaters is secret eating. Eat with others and enjoy their company!

8. **No distractions.** Don't eat in front of the TV, in the car, or while working. Be present when you're eating rather than distracted by something else. Bringing this awareness to your eating will also teach you to savor your food and eat slower. It helps to promote the opposite of the trancelike state that is one of the characteristics of binge eating.

9. **Clear your cupboards.** Decrease pitfalls and increase availability of booster foods in your home. If packaged foods are opened, it's too easy to say to yourself, "Oh well, it's open now, I have to finish it." Donate your packaged pitfalls to a homeless shelter and stock your shelves with healthy options.

10. **Lunch money.** If you worry about eating too much while out of the house, restrict how much money you carry and leave the credit card at home. If your lunch and snack at work is ten dollars, take just ten dollars with you.

11. **Hands off.** Don't taste when cooking. You'll be tempted into eating everything you've made. Just treat cooking your meal like a job. You're creating a healthy dinner for you or your family and you must complete the task without tasting it. If you really need an opinion, ask a friend or a family member to taste the food.

12. **Chew gum.** Chewing can be an anxiety reliever. So chew sugar-free gum to give your mouth something to do.

13. **Go public.** If you love a particular food and have avoided it because you're afraid it might trigger a binge, challenge this

belief by joining some friends and consuming one serving of the forbidden food. Forcing yourself to publicly enjoy a food you normally see as forbidden and secret can go a long way toward breaking its obsessive hold on you.

Freeing Yourself from Bingeing

The principles of Diet Rehab can help free you from a problematic relationship to food and from yo-yo dieting. If you are still experiencing binge eating after Diet Rehab, don't berate yourself. Instead, take what you have learned, and put those tools in your toolbox. Look at the continued bingeing as feedback that you may need to add another tool in the form of professional help. Find a mental health professional who specializes in disordered eating. If you need help, consult my website, www.drmikedow.com.

Where Do I Go from Here?

By now you have learned how to free yourself from some of the most common and addictive patterns people develop around eating. These tools will help you rehab your diet, which we're going to discuss in depth in the next section. Over the course of the next twenty-eight days you will finally be freeing yourself from craving the foods that keep you trapped in addiction.

PART IV

Rehab Your Diet

10

Change Your Tastes, Change Your Body

A few years ago, my patient Veronica was listing her long history with diets.

"When I did South Beach, I lost ten pounds in the first two weeks. Atkins was almost as good. And on the diet I did last year, I didn't lose ten pounds, but I did lose six." She looked at me hopefully. "So I'm hoping *your* program will be at least as good as those, Dr Mike."

I searched for the right questions to help her figure out the solution to this problem for herself. Finally, I said, "Veronica, how many diets have you been on in your life?"

"Oh, I don't know. Six? Ten? Maybe a dozen." She was frowning now.

"I see," I said. "And how many of them helped you keep the weight off?"

"Oh. Well." She sighed. "None of them, really. But that wasn't their fault. It was mine. I just couldn't stick to it. I'm always so bad at sticking to anything."

"Veronica," I said gently. "What if it wasn't your fault? What if it was that those diets just didn't give you the tools you needed to make the changes you were trying to make?"

To Veronica, this idea was a revelation. But that is the whole idea behind Diet Rehab: In order to give up the foods that are creating addictions and causing us to gain weight, we need the support of booster foods and activities, as well as booster mantras and attributes. When your life is full of foods and activities that support your brain chemistry, and when you're also allowing yourself at least some of your favorite treats, it's easy to let go of the pitfall foods that pull us into addiction.

There's one other thing we can do to support our transition from pitfalls to boosters: transform our tastes. Many of us have taught our taste buds to like only very sweet, salty, or fatty foods, making it difficult for us to appreciate the more subtle but equally delicious flavors to be found in fresh fruits, lightly cooked vegetables, and lean proteins. You *can* recalibrate your taste buds to like these "challenge foods," and I'll show you exactly how to do it—again, without your ever feeling deprived. You can even look forward to delicious all-booster versions that will start to taste *even better* than their pitfall food counterparts!

There are a couple of great outcomes that are possible here. One is that you may start to feel that the foods you used to love are simply too sweet, too salty, or too greasy. They might actually lose their appeal for you. This was the experience of people in a 1982 study who over a five-month period actually came to prefer less salty soups than they had in the beginning. Their palates had been successfully recalibrated.

Another possibility is that you'll love your old treats even more once they're a special break in your routine and not business as usual. Or perhaps some old treats won't make the cut, some will come to seem "just okay," and some will stand out as more delectable than ever, while you come to love your new "challenge foods."

Fortunately, you can recalibrate your palate at any age. Diabetics told to cut back on sugar often report that regular fruit tastes sweeter than it ever did before. The principle works the other way, too: The more we are exposed to a flavor, the more we get used to it and come to like it.

Whatever happens, you can expect a whole new world of tasting pleasure. So let's get started with the transformation, because this is definitely one of life's win-win situations!

Recalibration: My Own Story

When I developed my addiction to sweet and starchy foods, I didn't just transform my brain chemistry and increase my weight, I also reprogrammed my taste buds to respond only to super-sweet and super-salty tastes. I had "trained" them with doughnuts, sodas, and overly salted processed foods. In effect, I taught my taste receptors to set the preference bar very high for sweet and salt flavors and very low for natural, fresh flavors. I found nothing enticing about a nice, crisp salad garnished with cool cucumbers, sweet red and yellow peppers, and slightly sour red tomatoes. I wasn't in the least turned on by a serving of grilled asparagus splashed with lemon and a bit of extra-virgin olive oil, or by grilled salmon dressed with fresh dill. Sweet strawberries or tart raspberries didn't sound like a treat but like a consolation prize—what you were supposed to eat, not what you wanted to eat. Nothing registered as delicious if it wasn't "super-sweet" or "super-salty." I could barely taste anything that wasn't, let alone crave it.

Gradually, as my life filled up with serotonin booster activities, I was able to let go of some of my food addictions and make the transition to healthier food. But my mind was converted before my taste buds were. Even though I was a little concerned about my high cholesterol and had grown to dislike the constant spikes and crashes of a high-starch, high-sugar diet, I still thought sweets and starches tasted good, while my "challenge foods" of greens and fruits and lean proteins seemed bland and boring.

So I made the transition from pitfall to booster foods very, very gradually. One week I added a salad to my usual dinner of pasta and cheese. The next week I reduced the portion of pasta and added a vegetable. The following week I experimented with substituting fresh fruit for at least one of the three sugary desserts I ate throughout the day. The next week I started including lean protein as a main course at least once a day. Little by little, I filtered out most of the sweet, starchy, and salty foods and replaced them with fresh, healthy choices. And slowly—very slowly—I began to like my new menu, and even to actively look forward to it. Today I can honestly say that I *crave* a fresh salad at lunchtime. The succulent shrimp feels satisfying, the crisp, tart, Granny Smith apple wakes up the whole meal, and the light dressing of extra-virgin olive oil and tangy lemon makes everything taste genuinely delicious. Sure, sometimes I sub in some fries or a bowl of pasta. But most days I really *want* the salad. I've both let go of my addiction and recalibrated my taste buds. Now that I'm here, I can feel how positive reinforcement—my body looking better, my cholesterol in the normal range—helps me to keep going. And it feels effortless.

Natural Flavors

Whenever I lose interest in a food that I once used to crave, I remember that we were actually designed to eat what's good for us—we simply need reminding of what that tastes like. Our current taste buds are a mix of both inherited preferences and learned tastes—a combination of what ancient humans learned to prefer and what our high-fat, high-sugar diet has taught our taste buds to desire.

Interestingly, ancient humans developed flavor preferences as a means of survival, and we still share some of their tastes. Sweetness was appealing because ripe fruit was rich in vitamins. As our bodies learned it was safe and good to eat nourishing berries, apples, mangos, and pears, we learned to like those tastes. Similarly, we developed a dislike for bitterness, since that is the flavor of most natural poisons and food that has turned rancid. Pregnant women have a heightened ability to detect bitterness, which might have been a defense against exposing the unborn child to possible toxins.

Our early ancestors also contributed to our current taste for fatty foods, since in a world of scarcity, fat was a vital source of energy and a way to store calories when food was hard to find. Our current food supply not only is more readily available but also is littered with options that are far sweeter and richer in fat than the provisions our ancestors were eating. But we were never meant to be so overexposed to them. As a result, we no longer need to listen to our hardwired impulses to seek out sweet, fatty foods and to eat as much as possible whenever we can.

If you're reading these words before adding any boosters to your life, they may have the cold, ominous ring of a prison sentence. You may feel that I'm condemning you to a miserable, constricted life of either bland, uninteresting food or overwhelming, bitter, too-intense food. Or you may fear that I'm trying to deprive you of some of the few comforts left to you in a stressful, challenging time.

Believe me, I know what that feels like! But for the moment, please take it on faith that you *can* recalibrate your palate, just as I did, and it won't be either dreary or unpleasant—it will ultimately be both delicious and fun. We won't be eating exactly as our ancestors have programmed us to, but we won't be completely prey to modern fast-food and processed-food supplies either. Instead, we'll be making healthy choices that satisfy our ancient tastes while intelligently responding to our modern circumstances.

Are You a Supertaster?

Roughly one quarter of all humans are born with extra taste buds, a category known in nutritional science as "supertasters." Supertasters experience flavors more intensely—coffee is more bitter, sugar is intensely sweeter, chile is hotter.

Supertasters may love food more than most—American celebrity chef and talk-show host Rachael Ray, for example, is a supertaster, but she also gradually recalibrated her taste buds over years growing up in a Sicilian family that cooked with lots of booster foods. However, most supertasters tend to have trouble with such strong, bitter flavors as grapefruit, green tea, coffee, many vegetables, and some spices. As a group, they are incredibly sensitive to bitterness and taste it where others cannot. We don't know why some people are born supertasters and others are not, but being one affects the way you eat and can prove to be a challenge for those who want to change their diet.

Supertasters usually find the bland foods they feel comfortable with and stick with them, often choosing an "all-beige" diet of potatoes, pasta, fries, and bread. Supertasters like salt, too, since saltiness is one flavor that can counteract bitterness. If you're a supertaster who didn't grow up eating strong-flavored fresh fruits and vegetables, you may have some difficulty getting used to these new tastes. The solution for supertasters is the same as the rest of us: recalibrating taste buds by adding more and more booster foods to your everyday life. Knowing you're a supertaster helps you to understand why you have avoided healthier foods and gravitated toward an "all-beige" diet. For parents of children and teens who are picky eaters, it can help you to understand your child may have a genetic condition which may make it harder for him or her to accept new foods; it is not simply an act of rebellion or being stubborn. Supertasters will need to be particularly diligent and patient in recalibrating their taste buds. They will also benefit from the recalibration tools that follow.

To test whether you are, in fact, a supertaster, you can order a test on my website, www.drmikedow.com.

How to Transform Your Palate: Recalibration Made Easy

- **Mix a new food with a favorite one.** Try mixing some steamed broccoli into mac and cheese, or throw some lightly sautéed onions and peppers onto your burger. If you hate the idea of the new food, start with a tiny portion and gradually increase it. With bitter-flavored veggies, start by drizzling them with a honey-sweetened dressing that you gradually cut back or dipping them in ranch dressing, again reducing the amounts over time. Start with a dessert-spoonful per half-plate of veggies or salad, and work your way down from there. If you're not a cook, you can start with frozen, microwaveable packs of broccoli and cheese, Brussels sprouts, corn, or peas in butter sauce. Another useful trick is to chop or grate your vegetables very fine and stir them into a tomato-based sauce. It'll still taste like your favorite sauce and resemble it in texture. Gradually increase the size of the veggie pieces as you reduce the amount of sauce.

- **Think about the 4 Ts: taste, temperature, tint, and texture.** When my patients persistently have trouble trying something new, I talk them through the four Ts. If we separate the more daunting foods into these manageable categories, we can begin to approach them without fear. The key is to take the Ts one at a time. Going from sweet, hot, beige, chewy pizza to bitter, cold, green, and crisp salad may prove to be overwhelming, and then you may proclaim that you just don't like salads! Let's say you're struggling with taking even a bite of broccoli because the crunch and texture make you cringe. Start with a pureed broccoli soup (preferably low-salt or homemade), so that you don't have to deal with the new taste and the new texture at the same time. Once you've adjusted to the flavor, you can try eating the vegetable whole. If you struggle more with tint and temperature and don't like cold, green vegetables, grate or puree one or two stalks of broccoli into a hot marinara sauce. As you become used to a little bit of the taste, you can then change the temperature and try a small bite of broccoli in a cold pasta salad.

- **Use the Oreo technique.** Create a "sandwich" around your challenge food by taking a bite of a favorite food, then a bite of the new food, and then once again a bite of the first. Beginning and ending with a familiar food will help you to associate the challenge food with something delicious and comforting.

Take Your Time!

Remember, it usually takes at least ten exposures to a new food before you start to enjoy it and experience it as comfort food, so be patient with yourself. For supertasters, this number may be closer to thirty or forty.

Feeling Full: The Science of Satiety

Satiety is the quality of feeling full, or sated. The word "satisfied" comes from the same root and means essentially the same thing. By this point it probably won't surprise you to learn that satiety is both an emotional and biological function. In other words, we may feel hungry until we get the taste, the texture, or the eating experience that reminds us of our childhood or that somehow creates comfort for us. But we may also feel hungry—or dissatisfied—for biological reasons.

People who have food addictions or who are overweight often don't *feel* full even when they've eaten plenty of food. They feel driven to keep eating, usually to get the serotonin or dopamine boosters that are lacking in their diets and their lives. One of our goals with Diet Rehab is to keep you feeling satisfied all the time, so that emotional hunger and brain chemistry deprivation don't have to drive you to eat.

Now, here's a fact that will probably surprise you. I know I was astonished when I discovered it: High-fat and high-sugar food has what food scientists call a *low satiety* value. That is, your stomach gets almost no physical feeling of satisfaction and a very fleeting sense of fullness when you eat it. High-fat, high-sugar foods actually leave your stomach more quickly than booster foods, and the portions are smaller than the equivalent number of calories of booster foods. That means that all calories are *not* created equal, and figuring out how to feel satisfied and nourished is *not* a simple equation of just measuring how many calories you intake per day. The dark-chocolate-chip granola bar or baked sweet potato fries will actually leave you feeling full for longer than the candy bar or bag of crisps—even if the caloric contents of the two foods are the same.

Significantly, the more a food tends to tap into your addiction, flooding your brain with neurochemicals and burning out your receptors, the lower satiety value it is likely to have. The reverse is also true: The more stable a source of brain-balancing neurochemicals a food is, the more likely it is to be of high-satiety value.

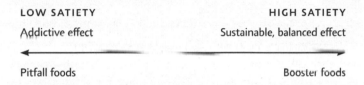

LOW SATIETY	HIGH SATIETY
Addictive effect	Sustainable, balanced effect
Pitfall foods	Booster foods

As we have seen, some pitfall foods give you a quick burst of dopamine, the pleasure chemical that is produced by a jolt of cocaine as well as by sex, desire, gambling, and physical thrills. For food companies, this is great news, since the consumer comes back consistently to the addictive sodas, crisps, candies, and pastries that are sold by the millions and billions, not to mention the addictive—and profit-making—appeal of all those foods loaded with "stealth" sugar and high-fructose corn syrup.

Luckily for Diet Rehab, booster foods have a high-satiety value. You'll be less likely to experience cravings if you can tune in to that feeling of fullness in your stomach—which becomes possible once your brain chemistry has been supported with adequate serotonin and dopamine.

Kitchen Kindness: Rehabbing Your Home

I think we've already established that I eat cookies, crisps, ice cream, and cake, not to mention the occasional bowl of mac and cheese. I eat them, I enjoy them, and I don't plan to give them up.

However, I don't keep them in my kitchen. I want to keep my sugary, starchy treats as enjoyable "food vacations"—not as daily staples. So instead of pitfalls, I stock lots of booster foods! Apples, grapes, bananas, baby carrots, and frozen berries can be found in my kitchen at all times. Buy some incredibly simple kitchen tools—for example, a mister that you can fill with extra-virgin olive oil. If there's no butter in the fridge, the whole family will start to spray this flavorful booster food to moisten whole-wheat bread or even popcorn. Invest in a capsule-based espresso machine for $99 (if you're like me, you will recoup your investment in just a few months by cutting back on your $4 lattes). I always keep decaf vanilla-flavored espresso capsules stocked. Or try some flavored decaf coffee or teas. They make for a delicious dessert while telling your body that the eating for the day has come to an end.

While you're stocking up on all these booster foods, set yourself up for success by doing a pitfall food raid on your kitchen. There's no sense in derailing your new plan with unnecessary temptation. Not having pitfall foods around all the time means they'll be even more special if you decide to treat yourself. All these kitchen fixes are simple to make and will boost not only your own health but the health of those in your household.

Once you've pitfall-proofed your kitchen, making positive choices in your own home will be much easier. But eating in a restaurant can be much trickier. The key is to be mindful of your options and to decrease the number of temptations. For example, I try to send back the basket of bread that is often brought to the table. I don't want to mindlessly reach for this treat food, and I don't want to feel compelled to eat it. Not having it easily available is part of my strategy for not relapsing into food addiction. When at buffets, I scope the entire selection before putting any food on my plate. And now that I've recalibrated my taste buds, there's nothing I crave more than a black decaf Americano to end a great meal. If I want a sweet treat, I have a frozen banana when I get home!

Finding the Time, Money, and Energy to Rehab Your Diet

"These frozen pies are just a few bucks and the family loves them."
"I don't have time to cook!"
"My kids only eat the stuff they see on TV."
"I can't afford to eat organic."

If shopping, cooking, and supplying yourself with high-quality food seems daunting—and if getting your family to change their tastes feels even more so—believe me, I understand. My mom was the same way: stressed out, busy, and forced to manage on a very tight budget. Between coping with my brother's medical issues and running her own business, cooking, shopping, and worrying about nutrition were the last things on her mind. We got by on pasta, crisps, and soda. If only we had known then what I have learned since: There are lots of quick, easy, and affordable ways to make healthy, delicious meals that even a picky kid will eat. Finger-sized munchies like baby carrots or cherry tomatoes dipped in hummus or salsa can easily replace crisps and candy. Keep washed grapes in the fridge and freezer at all times. Learn how to cook a few healthy one-pot meals like low-fat turkey chili that can be frozen. Swap white pasta with whole-wheat. Double vegetable-based pasta sauce and halve the noodles. Add broccoli to macaroni and cheese. When your bananas are turning a little black, peel and wrap in plastic wrap and throw them in the freezer.

Let me tell you up front: I'm busy, too, and though I love to eat, I don't especially like to cook. Nothing I make ever takes longer than twenty minutes. Sometimes I grill three lunches' worth of wild salmon and quinoa at one time or make a week's worth of veggie chili so that I only have to reheat it and prepare my vegetables. (For a look at my favorite recipes, see page 297; for answers to questions about Diet Rehab, see page 236 in Chapter 14.) I am living, breathing proof that you can eat well and easily—and if I can do it, anybody can!

Family Food

I understand your concerns about cost, but I promised you that while packaged foods *look* cheaper, you'll actually get more food for your money if you buy fresh foods and cook them. Your family will also start to snack less as their cravings for cookies and crisps diminish. And you might be surprised at how readily your kids will take to sweet crunchy carrots or tangy hummus or apples, raisins, and almonds as healthy snacks.

If you're worried about paying for organic, pick and choose. The most important foods to buy organic are the ones most exposed to pesticides and other pollutants when grown conventionally: strawberries, leafy green vegetables, apples, and carrots. The least important are the fruits with thick protective skins, such as bananas, citrus fruits, and avocados. I strongly recommend buying either organic milk or milk without the extra hormones.

It's also true that living on a healthy diet, at a healthy weight, means you are—well, healthier! Your immune system is stronger, your stamina is greater, and you'll face fewer doctor bills and days home from work.

But don't take my word for it. As you slowly but surely make the transition to healthy eating, you'll have a chance to see for yourself how much better you feel on a diet rich in booster foods and a life abundant in booster activities. Take your gradual detox one step at a time, and discover a whole new world of delicious foods, feeling full, and enjoying your healthy new body.

11

Salt Junkies: Hooked on the Gateway Drug

Whether we need serotonin, dopamine, or both, we all tend to love salty food. Why shouldn't we? It's stirred into just about every processed food there is—even the sweet ones! It's the cheap, easy additive that fast-food companies pour into their products to make it taste more intense, more flavorful, and more compelling. Once your taste buds get revved up on salt, it's hard for them to be satisfied with gentler, subtler flavors, and so we turn to overly sweet and fatty foods.

Our bodies require some natural salt, but the amount we actually need is tiny in comparison to the average person's intake. Other spices could be adding a kick to your food and improving your health at the same time, such as black pepper, cinnamon, rosemary, turmeric (found in curry powder and mustard), and capsaicin-packed spicy chiles.

In his 2009 book *The End of Overeating*, David Kessler, M.D., interviewed a former employee of Frito-Lay. The interviewee revealed that snack companies develop products that purposely trigger our addictive behaviors for sugar and fat, deliberately employing a technique called "layering," which puts fat and salt and sugar together to intensify the flavors of each. That's why I call salt the gateway drug. It sets us up for addictive relationships to serotonin and dopamine-flooding foods by cuing our taste buds to want only overwhelming and artificial flavors. Once our taste buds are ramped up to want extreme flavors, we crave super-sweet and super-fatty foods that then create addictions.

The Perils of Salt

Salt raises our blood pressure and causes dehydration. Besides potentially creating cardiovascular problems, dehydration causes us to eat more when what we really crave is water. Instead, we tend to snack on salty treats and processed foods, and then quench our thirst with sodas. Since sodas and other caffeinated drinks are diuretic, they cause our bodies to lose still more liquid, so the dehydration continues.

Salt is known to cause early death through heart attack and stroke. In fact, salt is estimated to be killing about 100,000 people each year. That's the equivalent of a wide-body 767 airliner of people crashing and dying every day.

Breaking the Habit: Jasmine's Story

My patient Jasmine ran into problems with salt when she tried to give herself a new food regime. A single woman in her mid-thirties, Jasmine worked long hours as a public-interest lawyer. She'd grab a latte and Danish as she rushed to work in the morning. A few hours later, she'd crash and need another coffee and maybe a bagel with cream cheese from the office snack bar. She'd skip lunch, but she always got hungry around three p.m., when she would ravenously snack on something salty, such as crisps or pretzels. She'd have a slice of pizza around seven p.m. When she finally got home at ten or eleven, she'd throw some pasta into a pot of boiling water and serve it up to herself with some creamy Alfredo sauce or oily white clam sauce from the grocery store.

As Jasmine and I worked together, she began to realize that her eating habits fed her sugar/starch and fat addictions in problematic ways. But she still didn't have time to cook, and so she switched to what she thought were healthy frozen meals. What she didn't realize, though, was that this was yet another processed food with a salt content just as alarming as some of her previous go-to foods.

Eventually, Jasmine found that she could just as easily throw together a healthy salad or low-salt, low-fat soups and stews that she could make for the week and put in the freezer, thawing them out when she wanted them. Avoiding her addictions was a lot about planning for Jasmine, since she was so time-constrained. She was shocked at how much more easily her hunger was satisfied and how cutting back on salt changed her eating habits.

She began waking up earlier, feeling less sluggish than before. She was up in time to make a healthy breakfast of fruit and yogurt or oatmeal, which kept her feeling full until her lunch of grilled chicken salad or whatever lighter option she felt like having.

Without salt, Jasmine was able to steer herself away from sweet, starchy, and fatty foods far more easily. It took a while for her sense of taste to adjust, but once it did she was amazed.

"I can't believe how good everything tastes!" she told me. "I had almonds with no added salt yesterday. They would have tasted like cardboard to me before, but now they're delicious! They've got so much flavor and they kept me full until dinner."

Jasmine lost seven pounds in three weeks. Cutting the salt had been the clincher for her.

"The first few days of low salt were tough," she admitted. "But then I felt like I was hardly even trying. I really started enjoying food, instead of just feeling starved or stuffed."

Stealth Salt

It's almost impossible to keep your salt intake down if you eat any processed or fast food. Like sugar, it's hidden everywhere. Some restaurant entrees have 2,000 milligrams or more in a single dish—far more than the maximum suggested daily allowance of 1,500 milligrams for people over fifty-one, African-Americans, or those with high blood pressure, diabetics, or chronic kidney disease. For people not in these groups, that one entrée alone is dangerously close to the daily recommended allowance of 2,300 milligrams. Burgers typically contain more than 1,000 milligrams. Canned and restaurant soups can also be huge salt-packers.

Salt is hidden in most packaged food items, including cookies and cakes, as most food companies use salt to preserve their products. Accordingly, pasta sauces, broths, lunch meats, salad dressings, cheeses, crackers, and frozen foods are frequently swimming in salt.

The Problem with Packaged Meals: Andrew's Story

Andrew came to me at age fifty after being diagnosed with high blood pressure. He was really shaken when his doctor had prescribed hypertension medication because his father had died of a heart attack at the relatively young age of fifty-five, while his grandfather had suffered a debilitating stroke. Andrew was suddenly terrified that this was his future, too.

From the outside, Andrew appeared quite healthy. He did some moderate exercise three times a week and was perhaps only ten pounds overweight. He insisted he ate at home and avoided fast food.

"I don't even eat that much anyway," he sighed. "I do love tortilla chips, and I always have pretzels when I watch a game at the bar, but

I almost never eat fast food and I barely ever have a drink! How has this happened to me?" He was visibly upset.

I suggested that Andrew write down everything he ate in detail for a week. At his next appointment I was able to see the problem immediately: It wasn't just his once-a-week pretzel habit or the occasional treat of tortilla chips. Andrew was living on packaged TV dinners—and they were simply saturated in salt.

As a bachelor, Andrew didn't see the point of cooking for himself, so he stocked up on reasonably sized frozen dinners of roast beef and potatoes, chicken with vegetables, and premixed noodle dishes. He had trained his taste buds to expect strong, salty flavors, so he found himself sprinkling extra salt on his sandwiches at lunch and craving bacon at breakfast time. Andrew was so careful to avoid overeating that he had evaded a fat addiction—but at 4,000 milligrams per day, his salt intake was off the charts.

Now Andrew carefully reads the labels on everything at the grocery store. He doesn't buy anything with more than 500 milligrams of sodium per serving. He's learned to cook some basic meals from scratch and recalibrated his taste buds, so that fresh foods and alternate flavors now seem more satisfying than his old, processed diet.

"Now I can taste the salt in things too much," Andrew laughs. "If I find myself at a restaurant with friends, the soup especially always tastes disgusting to me now. So salty! I don't even think about those pretzels and crisps anymore. Sometimes I'll have unsalted popcorn, but that's about the only snack I like now."

Andrew wasn't just enjoying new, fresh flavors, he was experiencing a dopamine high from trying new things. He was also feeling increased self-esteem from learning to cook for himself—he even joined a cooking class, where he made a few new friends. Meanwhile, his blood pressure has fallen to a normal level, and he feels a sense of optimism that is giving him the confidence to keep making changes.

Hypertension Horrors

- Every American over fifty has a 90 percent chance of developing hypertension, which increases the risk of heart disease and stroke.
- If you're overweight, eating processed food, and doing little physical activity, you are the most likely type to develop this condition.
- Hypertension is preventable through salt reduction, exercise, and maintaining a healthy body weight.

Keys to Cutting Salt

- **Read all labels.** Limit your intake of anything with over 500 milligrams of salt per serving.
- **Wean yourself off the taste.** Start by slowly reducing your salt intake, then keep reducing, little by little. Give your taste buds a chance to recalibrate themselves. (For more on recalibrating your tastes, see Chapter 10.)
- **Cook for yourself.** When you do, replace salt with strong, stimulating flavors such as turmeric, rosemary, balsamic or apple cider vinegar, ginger, lemon, lime, cracked black pepper, hot chile peppers, onions, and garlic.
- **Experiment.** Play with adding new herbs and spices to your diet. Try cooking foods from different countries, or create some new versions of old comfort foods.
- **Avoid overwhelming a dish with too many seasonings.** Learn to appreciate the subtle flavors that make food worth tasting.

Exploring New Flavors: Brian's Story

Adding hot sauce to food was a useful helper for my patient Brian, a moderately obese man who used to add salt to everything he ate, including his favorite high-fat foods that were already brimming with hidden salt. When I suggested he try to substitute hot sauce for salt, Brian agreed to give it a try. Although the hot sauce contained a small amount of salt, it was a far healthier choice than the previous alternative. Brian just needed to know he could rely on a strong taste that wasn't salt.

Eventually, Brian got tired of everything tasting of Tabasco and switched to other spices and herbs to flavor his food. He no longer missed his salt, and cutting down on it freed him to let go of his addiction to high-fat food. He's now lost half his target weight.

Flavor Your Food Without Salt

Ever wonder which flavors go with what? Here are some tips to get you started on flavorful no-salt cooking:

HERBS AND SPICES

Basil: Italian foods, such as tomatoes, pasta, chicken, fish, and shellfish

Bay leaf: bean or meat stews and soups

Chili powder: bean or meat stews and soups

Chives: sauces, soups, baked potatoes, salads, omelets, pasta, seafood, and meat

Coriander: Mexican, Latin American, and Asian cuisine; rice, beans, fish, shellfish, poultry, vegetables, salsas, and salads

Cumin: curried vegetables, poultry, fish, and beans

Curry: Indian or southeast Asian cuisine; lamb or meat-based dishes and soups

Dill: seafood, chicken, yogurt, cucumbers, green beans, tomatoes, potatoes, and beetroot

Ginger: chicken, rice, and marinades

Oregano: Italian and Greek cuisine; meat and poultry dishes

Paprika: Spanish dishes, potatoes, soups, stews, baked fish, and salad dressings

Rosemary: mushrooms, roasted potatoes, stuffing, ripe melon, poultry, and meats

Sage: poultry stuffing, chicken, duck, pork, aubergine, and bean stews and soups

Tarragon: chicken, veal, fish, shellfish, eggs, salad dressings, tomatoes, mushrooms, and carrots

Thyme: Fish, shellfish, poultry, tomatoes, beans, aubergine, mushrooms, potatoes, and summer squash

Turmeric: Indian cuisine

For some suggestions on how to actually use these spices, see Appendix A for my favorite quick-and-easy recipes. Also check out my website, www.drmikedow.com, for some of my favorite resources for recipes and cooking tips.

When to Add the Herbs

Put in dried herbs early when cooking, but toss in fresh herbs at the end. That way, the intense taste of the dried herbs can work its way through the food, but the fresh herbs will still taste fresh.

Start Slow . . . But Keep Going

Like everything else we've talked about, changing your salt intake is so much more about what we add than what we take away. The point here is not to shackle yourself to a low-sodium diet; it's to embark on an adventurous high-on-every-herb-and-spice-other-than-salt diet! Adding booster activities to your life (found on pages 208 and 223) means that your life will be filled with so many other kicks—such as the thrill of finally beating your kids at Monopoly or the pleasure of that spa day you've given yourself—that frozen pot pies will start to taste like what they are: salt-laden, fat-dripping, artery-clogging expendables for a life that is rich in so many other ways.

12

Starved for Serotonin: Jonesing for Sugar and Carbs

id you find out in Chapter 4 that you were starving for serotonin? If so, you're very likely in the grip of chronic anxiety. Sometimes it's just a little worry about having to pack for a weekend trip ("What if I forget my travel clock! What if I oversleep?"). Sometimes it's more significant dread about major deadlines or unpaid bills ("We could lose the house! The kids will have to leave their schools! I'm too old to get another job!"). Either way, if you're short on serotonin, life is one long series of unnerving challenges, and you're never completely sure that you'll be able to meet them—at least not to your own satisfaction.

Perhaps your serotonin shortage leads you into the seven pitfall thought patterns (see page 53), in which anxious, obsessive, or pessimistic thoughts seem to take over your mind and your feelings. Suddenly you're locked into a downward spiral of anxiety, which depletes your serotonin, which makes you more anxious, which further depletes your serotonin . . .

Following are some typical worries that my serotonin-starved patients share with me. Do any of these anxiety-provoking thoughts sound familiar?

- Other people have it easier than me. Their lives are more together.
- I'm so fat. Everyone is thinner than I am.
- No one else has to think about every single bite—but I do, or I'll gain a ton. What is *wrong* with me?
- My weight is so out of control. My job is probably in danger too. And I'll never have a good relationship!

I wish I could reassure you that everyone has moments of feeling insecure, unattractive, and out of control—it is by no means just you. I wish I could reassure you, too, that your worries are not reliable guides to reality but only to the place where your mind and feelings go when you are starving for serotonin. Is it any wonder that you crave the comfort foods that help to boost your serotonin levels? You are simply trying to raise your serotonin levels by looking for sweets and simple carbs to ease your anxiety and give you at least a temporary infusion of calm. If you're short on serotonin, you're likely to gravitate toward foods made with processed sugar and white flour: cakes, cookies, pasta, bread. Our goal is to help you find all the calm and comfort you deserve—but from healthier foods and activities.

Your Diet Rehab Treatment Plan

When you start your 28-day Diet Rehab, you'll be nourishing your mind, body, and spirit with serotonin booster foods and activities. Think about loading yourself up with the following "S" words:

- Sweet—Berries and other fruits can give you a boost of sweetness that can ease your cravings for processed sugar. They produce a slow and steady boost of serotonin in your brain and won't spike blood sugar the way candy or white starches will.

- Starchy—Switch up your starches. Brown rice, whole-grain cereals, and sprouted breads have a high satiety value, which, as we discussed in Chapter 10, means that you'll feel fuller for longer and by eating less. These foods also give you a more prolonged serotonin boost than foods made with white flour. Check out my favorite quick-and-easy recipes in Appendix A for suggestions of meals made up entirely of serotonin boosters, or look at the booster snacks and swaps on pages 243 and 246.
- Stretch—Choose calming exercises like yoga, Pilates, and simple daily stretching to cue your body to make more serotonin. Deep breathing, relaxing baths, and taking some quiet time are also great options. You can even use your serotonin booster foods to create a soothing experience—sip some chamomile tea while reading in bed or make a Greek yogurt and fruit smoothie to enjoy after an afternoon stroll.
- Sleep—Did you know your body releases more ghrelin—the "hunger" hormone—when you don't get your seven or eight hours every night? Lack of sleep also interferes with your body's production of serotonin. A big mistake many of my patients make is falling asleep with the computer or television on. Their lights can actually disrupt your circadian rhythms, which promote healthy sleeping and eating patterns, so unplug the electronics and sleep your way to weight loss!
- Sun—The relaxing rays of warm sunshine can have a powerful serotonin-boosting effect. Twenty minutes of sunlight gives you a healthy boost of vitamin D, a booster that helps combat depression. Don't overdo it, though. Twenty minutes a day of being outside is enough to feel the benefit.
- Soothing—The fragrance of lavender incense, the warmth of a crackling fire, and the peaceful calm of a walk can boost your

serotonin levels, as can a relaxing massage, a long bath, or a comforting talk with a friend.

- Spiritual—Reconnecting to your life's purpose and feeling your place in the universe can breed a sense of peace and security like nothing else. Let your longing for serotonin remind you that your spiritual side is hungry, too. Find your own relationship to prayer, secular meditation, time in nature, or volunteer activities that allow you to experience your deepest connection with our planet and our world.

Serotonin Booster Foods

The first step in your Diet Rehab plan is adding some of these serotonin booster foods to your diet. Look over this list. There are bound to be at least a few foods that you already like. If plain yogurt with some organic blueberries and a cup of white tea sounds like an appetizing snack, then that could be one of the first boosters you swap in. As the weeks go on, you can try to experiment with serotonin booster foods you've never had, such as lentils and quinoa with balsamic vinegar and a sprinkling of olive oil and oregano. You can also look back to pages 199–200 for some great suggestions on pairing herbs with foods, and check out my favorite quick-and-easy recipes in Appendix A. Be patient with yourself, and remember, the more you try it, the better the chance is you'll come to crave it.

What About Portion Sizes?

Feel free to enjoy generous but reasonable portion sizes of booster foods. The good news is that without excessive pitfall foods hijacking your brain chemistry, you will actually begin to sense when you need to eat and how much will be based on actual physical hunger. For a few booster foods, such as olive oil and nuts, I've provided guidelines, but for the rest, just eat what you like in reasonable amounts. In general, booster foods help you to recalibrate your taste buds to prefer generous servings of whole fruits, vegetables, and lean proteins with reasonable servings of whole grains. I have never treated a food addict or even a binge eater who had a problem eating too many whole fruits and vegetables! Most people will find that as they add new, exciting booster foods, they will experience a significant decrease in their desire for packaged pitfall snacks, which are usually mostly unhealthy carbohydrates and fats.

LOW-FAT DAIRY/DAIRY ALTERNATIVES

- almond milk, unsweetened
- any nonfat or reduced-fat cheese
- fat-free cream cheese
- low-fat cottage cheese
- low-fat goat's milk
- nonfat or low-fat kefir
- nonfat or low-fat sour cream
- plain low-fat Greek yogurt
- plain low-fat soy yogurt
- plain low-fat yogurt
- skim or 1% milk

WHOLE GRAINS AND SEEDS

- barley
- brown rice
- buckwheat
- flaxseed
- high-fiber bars (at least 5 grams of fiber per serving)
- high-fiber tortilla (at least 3 grams of fiber per serving)
- plain instant oatmeal
- quinoa
- soba noodles
- spelt
- coarse-cut oats
- whole-grain bread/bagel/pita (at least 3 grams of fiber per serving)
- whole-grain cereal (at least 5 grams of fiber per serving)
- whole-wheat pasta

PROTEIN: UNFRIED AND UNBREADED

- Animal protein
  - eggs
  - chicken
  - poussin
  - turkey, ground turkey, turkey bacon
- Seafood: favor wild-caught over farm-raised
  - clams
  - halibut
  - herring
  - mackerel
  - salmon
  - sardines
  - scallops
  - shrimp
  - sole
  - trout
  - tuna
  - white fish
- Beans
  - adzuki beans
  - black beans
  - black-eyed peas
  - cannellini beans
  - chickpeas
  - edamame
  - fava beans
  - great northern beans
  - hummus
  - cannellini beans
  - kidney beans
  - lentils
  - lima beans
  - mung beans
  - haricot beans
  - toor dal
  - pinto beans
  - refried beans: fat-free only, no hydrogenated oils
  - soybeans
  - soy nuts
  - split peas
  - tempeh
  - tofu
  - white beans
  - yuba (dried bean curd skin)
- Nuts and seeds: just 10 to 15 per serving, favor plain and unsalted
  - almond and other nut butters
  - almonds
  - cashews
  - hazelnuts
  - peanut butter (natural)
  - pecans
  - pistachios
  - sunflower seeds
  - walnuts
- Other protein sources
  - casein protein
  - soy crisps
  - soy protein
  - whey protein

VEGETABLES: RAW, GRILLED, SAUTÉED, STEAMED, OR JUICED

- aubergine
- beetroot
- bell peppers
- broccoli
- Brussels sprouts
- cabbage
- carrots
- celery
- collard greens
- kale
- mushrooms
- mustard greens
- onions
- popcorn: air-popped or microwaved (low-fat, no hydrogenated oils)
- romaine lettuce
- seaweeds
- spinach
- squash
- sweet potatoes
- Swiss chard
- tomatoes
- turnip greens
- yams

FRUITS: UNSWEETENED (NO SUGAR, SYRUP, OR OIL ADDED), NOT JUICED, WHOLE FRUIT

- açaí berries
- apples
- apricots
- bananas
- blueberries
- cantaloupe
- cherries
- cranberries
- figs
- goji berries
- grapefruit
- grapes
- kiwis
- lemons
- limes
- olives
- oranges
- papayas
- pears
- plantains
- plums
- prunes
- raspberries
- strawberries

OILS

- extra-virgin olive oil (for dressings)
- virgin olive oil (for cooking)

SPICES AND HERBS: FAVOR SOOTHING AND FAMILIAR

- basil
- cinnamon
- cloves
- cumin
- dill
- ginger
- oregano
- parsley
- peppermint
- rosemary
- sage
- thyme

DRINKS AND DESSERTS

- unsweetened tea: herbal, white, red, or decaf
- unsweetened decaf coffee
- hot water with lemon
- sparkling water with a splash of fruit juice
- vegetable juice
- dark chocolate with at least 70% cacao
- frozen plain bananas
- frozen plain berries

Serotonin Booster Activities

Through the twenty-eight days of Diet Rehab, you'll also be adding booster activities to your daily life. Since low serotonin means high anxiety, be kind and gentle with yourself when deciding which activities on this list to try. Start out with those that sound pleasurable and easy. Once you've got your serotonin stabilized, some of the more challenging options here may no longer feel like they're out of reach. As this happens, you may discover some of your own favorite serotonin booster activities. Just remember: Slow and steady wins the race!

Adopt a rescue animal
Apologize

Arrange an outing to a movie or concert
Ask your barista how his or her day is
Ask a stressed coworker if there's something you can do to help
Attend a 12-step meeting
Attend a class
Attend a religious service or Bible study
Balance your checkbook
Be honest
Become a Guide/Scout volunteer, or join a youth mentoring
    programme
Bird watch
Bowl
Breathe deeply for five minutes
Bring a reusable bag to the store
Bring home one flower for your significant other . . . or yourself
Build a sand castle
Build a snowman
Call just to say, "I love you"
Canoe
Coach a kid's team
Cook
Cuddle with your significant other or pet
Do a crossword puzzle
Do a favor and expect nothing in return
Do the dishes
Do your errands on foot or on your bike
Do your taxes
Eat dinner in the dark and taste every bite
Exercise
Fly a kite
Forgive
Garden
Get health insurance

Get or give a massage
Get rid of clutter
Get that mammogram or medical test you've been putting off
Give somebody a compliment
Give your pet a bath
Give yourself a compliment
Give yourself a face mask or scrub
Go a whole day without using your car
Go dancing
Go fishing
Go online and look at photos of foreign cities or landscapes
Go to a farmers' market
Go to a library or bookstore to just browse
Go to a museum
Go to a petting zoo
Go to a stand-up comedy show
Go to bed thirty minutes earlier
Go to the opera or theater
Go to the top floor of a parking structure and take in the view
Golf
Half-smile for five minutes
Have a dance party with your kids
Have a good conversation
Have a TV- or computer-free evening
Hike a trail
Hold a baby
Hold a puppy
Hold hands
Hold the door for someone
Horseback ride
Hug somebody
Invite friends or family over just to chat
Jog

Join a support group

Journal—jot down what you're grateful for, any overwhelming feelings you'd like to unload, or any great ideas!

Kayak

Knit

Let the person with just a few things go ahead of you at the store

Light a candle or incense

Listen to a friend's problems

Listen to classical or peaceful music

Look at old pictures

Look in the mirror and find one thing you like about the way you look

Look into someone's eyes when you're talking to them

Make a five-dollar donation to a charity online

Make amends

Make love

Meditate (download my serotonin-boosting meditation at www .drmikedow.com)

Mow your lawn

Open a Facebook account and get in touch with an old friend

Open a savings account and plan for a trip you want to take

Organize your desk, closet, or junk drawer

Paint

Pamper yourself

Pay a bill

Pay for the person behind you at the tollbooth

Plan a potluck

Plan a surprise party

Plan for retirement

Play a game—with a team or by yourself

Play an instrument

Play with your pet

Practice tai chi/qi gong

Pray

Put on warm socks

Quilt

Rake the leaves

Read

Recycle

Rub lotion on your hands or feet

Sail

Say hello to a stranger in the elevator

Say no when you need to, and don't feel guilty about it

Scrapbook

Send a card

Send somebody flowers

Set the table and sit down to eat

Sing along to the radio

Skip rocks

Skype with a faraway friend

Smell the roses . . . literally

Smile

Speak your truth

Spend a little time at a park or beach

Start a piggy bank

Stop and admire the view

Stretch for five minutes or more

Study

Sunbathe (no more than twenty minutes or with sunblock)

Swim

Take a bath

Take a small step at achieving a big goal

Take a twenty-minute nap

Take a walk—a brisk after-work stress reliever or a leisurely after-dinner stroll. Get the family involved!

Take a yoga or Pilates class

Take deep breaths for several minutes while visualizing positive
thoughts

Take photos—even if it's just with your cell phone

Take some old clothes to a charity shop

Take the stairs

Talk to a therapist

Tell a friend how much he or she means to you

Tell yourself three things you like about yourself

Treat yourself to a subscription to your favorite magazine

Try bright light therapy in the morning

Try positive visualization

Turn off your phone for one hour

Visit a loved one's grave and tell them why they'd be proud of you
today

Volunteer

Walk or run for a cause

Walk your dog

Watch a funny or inspiring show on TV

Watch your favorite romantic comedy

Write a letter longhand, on paper

Write a poem

Write down your childhood dreams

Write your memoir

Serotonin Pitfall Foods

While you're stabilizing your serotonin booster foods and activities
in the weeks to come, you'll also need to be mindful of cutting back
on the following serotonin pitfalls. Not to worry, because your serotonin will become balanced through other, sustainable sources of this
feel-good chemical. When that happens, eating fewer of these pitfall

foods will start to feel effortless. When in doubt, check the label. The main culprits to be on the lookout for are high-fructose corn syrup, white flour, sugar, and any partially hydrogenated oils. These pitfall ingredients make what you'd expect to be a booster—such as some energy bars or "wheat" breads—a pitfall. However, most pitfall foods are fairly easy to spot. Here are some of the most common serotonin pitfall foods:

Breadsticks and crackers
Cake
Candy
Coffee with flavored syrup
Cookies
Doughnuts
Fruit juice
Hot chocolate
Ice cream
Jam/sweetened spreads
Milk chocolate
Muffins
Pancakes
Pie
Soda
Sugar (white, brown, powdered)
Sweetened breakfast cereals
Syrup
Waffles
Whipped cream
White bread
White flour
White pasta

One Step at a Time

So now you know *what* you need to do. If you're like most serotonin-deprived people, *how* you do it will be just as important in your transformation process. Be forgiving with yourself, and always be on the lookout for what you did *right* today as opposed to focusing on what you did *wrong*. Some low-serotonin perfectionists will want to bypass gradual detox and shock their brains right into an all-booster-food regime beginning on day one. Remember, this is probably the same perfectionism that has gotten you into trouble before!

When it comes to weight loss and changing your life, it's a marathon, not a sprint. And the race is only with yourself. Since food can be addictive, the same catchphrases that apply to other addictions apply: One day at time. Easy does it. Fake it till you make it. Since low serotonin can trigger feelings of perfectionism, self-criticism, and doubt, be on the lookout for those seven pitfall thought patterns (see page 53) trying to steer you off course. When you notice them, that's the perfect time to add one of the serotonin booster activities to your day to take your mind away from their destructive and seductive lure!

13

Dopamine-Deprived: Longing for Fat and Caffeine

I f you discovered in Chapter 5 that you're low on dopamine, you may
be frustrated with a life that seems too slow and boring, or you might
have the opposite problem: feeling overwhelmed by a life that feels too
fast and full. Maybe you bounce from deadline to deadline or crisis to
crisis, always pulling out a little more energy, a few more reserves—
only to feel burned out. Or perhaps you feel trapped in a dead-end job
or in a narrow life, wondering how you ended up spending every waking minute on child care and housekeeping, with so little room for fun.

If the serotonin-deficient food addict is an anxious eater, the
dopamine-deficient food addict is a depressed one. Feeling empty,
lonely, or perhaps a little bit lost can all lead to self-medicating with
high-fat, dopamine-rich foods. Plus, low-dopamine types are much more
likely to avoid talking about feelings than those with low serotonin, so
your friends may not know that you're unhappy or how frustrated and
unfulfilled you are. You may be missing the support of others who are
intimidated by your seemingly perfect life and your unwillingness to
ask for or accept help.

Even if your life looks successful and put together, your dopamine deprivation may reflect some subtle problems that you're having trouble acknowledging, even to yourself. Maybe you and your partner are too tired for the kind of sex you'd like to have. Maybe you've mastered your formerly satisfying job and no longer find it a challenge. Maybe your wonderful kids fill your heart with love—but still you long for a bit of adventure.

Either way, if you're dopamine-deprived, you are likely to crave genuine excitement to combat a growing sense of depression. Do any of the following thoughts and feelings sound familiar?

- Is this all there is?
- Surely life should hold more than this!
- Where did all the fun and excitement go?
- I haven't done anything new in a long time . . .
- I don't recognize myself—how did I become so boring?
- I used to be a passionate person—what happened?

I want to help you awaken that part of yourself that feels stifled and suppressed by either boredom or too much work. Hopefully the Diet Rehab program will convince you to make the time and energy for yourself, and to commit to the pleasure in your life as much as you have already committed to your daily tasks and duties. You'll see that high-fat foods, which trigger a short-term rush of dopamine, aren't adding any satisfaction to a life that might seem too stale. Our goal is to help you find all the thrills and adventure you crave—but from healthier foods and activities.

Your Diet Rehab Treatment Plan

When you start your 28-day Diet Rehab, you'll be nourishing your mind, body, and spirit with dopamine booster foods and activities. I want you to remind yourself of the following "D" words:

217

- Deep-fried-and-fatty to lean-and-mean: If you're like most dopamine-deprived people, you will have gravitated to french fries, fried chicken, and energy drinks to give you the spark that you were longing for in your life. But there's another great source of dopamine, and that's lean protein. If you're dopamine-deprived, you need protein—and lots of it. You should be sure to have some protein with every meal, and you need protein-rich snacks throughout the day to protect yourself against cravings. Check out Appendix A for some of my favorite quick and easy recipes for dopamine booster meals, or look at page 243 for some dopamine booster snacks. You'll see that tasty foods like apples and almond butter are a great way to get a dopamine fix.

- Daring: You're craving change, excitement, and adventure, so mix it up by learning a new skill or doing something you've always dreamed about doing. Ski down a mountain, learn to parasail, ride in a hot-air balloon, or do some public speaking. Sign up for that online dating service, or ask that cute barista out for breakfast. Scare the hell out of yourself! The more adventure in your life, the less fat you'll crave. Even mix up your dopamine booster foods in daring ways. Egg whites, grilled chicken breast, and broccoli in a homemade sauce of red bell peppers, jalapeños, and Tabasco sauce may sound daunting to some—but not for you!

- Delight: If we don't get delight in our lives, we'll look for it in our food. Marvel at a sunset, visit an intriguing new stretch of a neighborhood, spend ten minutes a day doing something that you love. You'll fill up on pleasure, and those french fries will just look like, well, greasy potatoes.

- Desire: I can't advise you to fall in love—but if you did, it would be great for your waistline! What about rekindling some romance with your significant other? Or, if you're single, do something you've always considered romantic, sexy, or thrilling: visit Italy, learn to play poker, take a tango class. Find *something* you desire, and give yourself permission to pursue it.

• Dare: Dopamine-deprived people need challenges, so test your creativity and see what you come up with. You might decide to redesign your garden, move around furniture in your living room or bedroom, or reorganize your closets. Learn a language, play competitive Scrabble, or just pick up a book of Sudoku—anything to experience a sense of struggle and accomplishment.

Dopamine Booster Foods

The first step in your plan is adding some of these dopamine booster foods to your diet. You don't have to eat all these foods, but if you could find ten or twenty you like, that'd be a great place to start. And since you're likely craving new adventures in your life, it won't be hard for you to try new foods. Maybe you could even challenge yourself by trying every food on this list. I dare you!

What About Portion Sizes?

Feel free to enjoy generous but reasonable portion sizes of booster foods. The good news is that without excessive pitfall foods hijacking your brain chemistry, you will actually begin to sense when you need to eat based on physical hunger and also when to stop. For a few booster foods, such as olive oil and nuts, I've provided guidelines, but for the rest, just eat what you like in reasonable portions. In general, booster foods help you to recalibrate your taste buds to prefer generous servings of whole fruits, vegetables, and lean proteins with some whole grains. I have never treated a food addict or even a binge eater who had a problem eating too many whole fruits and vegetables! Most people will find that as they add new, exciting booster foods, they will experience a significant decrease in their desire for packaged pitfall snacks, which are usually mostly unhealthy carbohydrates and fats.

LOW-FAT DAIRY/DAIRY SUBSTITUTES

- almond milk, unsweetened
- any nonfat or reduced-fat cheese
- fat-free cream cheese
- low-fat goat's milk
- nonfat or low-fat kefir
- nonfat or low-fat sour cream
- plain low-fat Greek yogurt
- skim or 1% milk

WHOLE GRAINS AND SEEDS

- flaxseed
- high-protein pasta, such as Barilla Plus
- quinoa

PROTEIN: UNFRIED AND UNBREADED

- animal protein
  - buffalo (5% or less fat)
  - chicken
  - poussin
  - eggs
  - elk (5% or less fat)
  - lamb shank or leg
  - lean beef (5% or less fat)
  - lean lamb (5% or less fat)
  - low-fat sliced ham
  - ostrich (5% or less fat)
  - pork
  - turkey, ground turkey, turkey bacon
  - venison (5% or less fat)

OTHER PROTEIN SOURCES

- casein protein
- protein bars (15 grams or more of protein)
- protein shakes with no added sugar
- whey protein

SEAFOOD: FAVOR WILD-CAUGHT OVER FARM-RAISED

- clams
- halibut
- herring
- mackerel
- oysters
- salmon
- sardines
- scallops
- shrimp
- sole
- trout
- tuna
- white fish

BEANS

- adzuki beans
- black beans
- black-eyed peas
- cannellini beans
- chickpeas
- edamame
- fava beans
- white beans
- hummus
- cannellini beans
- kidney beans
- lentils
- lima beans
- mung beans
- haricot beans
- toor dal
- pinto beans
- refried beans: fat-free only, no hydrogenated oils
- soybeans
- split peas
- white beans
- yuba (bean curd skin)

NUTS AND SEEDS: JUST 10 TO 15 PER SERVING; FAVOR PLAIN AND UNSALTED

- almond and other nut butters
- almonds
- Brazil nuts
- cashews
- hazelnuts
- macadamia nuts
- peanut butter (natural only; no hydrogenated oils)
- pecans
- pistachios
- pumpkin seeds
- sesame seeds
- sunflower seeds
- walnuts

VEGETABLES: RAW, GRILLED, SAUTÉED, STEAMED, OR JUICED;
UNLIMITED PORTIONS UNLESS OTHERWISE NOTED

- asparagus
- aubergine
- avocado (half; no guacamole)
- beetroot
- bell peppers
- broccoli
- Brussels sprouts
- cabbage
- carrots
- celery
- collard greens
- corn
- cucumbers
- fennel
- garlic
- green beans
- kale
- leeks
- mushrooms
- mustard greens
- onions
- popcorn: air-popped, microwave (low-fat, no hydrogenated oils) or stove-popped in rapeseed oil
- romaine lettuce
- seaweeds
- spinach
- squash
- Swiss chard
- tomatoes
- turnip greens

FRUITS: UNSWEETENED (NO SUGAR, SYRUP, OR OIL
ADDED), NOT JUICED, WHOLE FRUIT

- açaí berries
- bananas
- blueberries
- cranberries
- goji berries
- lemons
- limes
- olives
- raspberries
- strawberries

OILS AND DRESSINGS: HEAVY ON THE VINEGAR, LIGHT ON THE OIL

- rapeseed oil
- extra-virgin olive oil (for dressings)
- mustard
- trans-fat-free spreads like Smart Balance
- vinegar
- virgin olive oil (for cooking)

SPICES AND HERBS: FAVOR EXCITING AND NEW

- black pepper
- cayenne pepper
- chile pepper
- coriander
- dill
- ginger
- hot sauce
- low-fat mayonnaise
- mustard seeds
- oregano
- thyme
- turmeric (mustard)
- vinegar

DRINKS, DESSERTS, AND SWEETENERS

- unsweetened tea: green or black
- unsweetened iced tea
- unsweetened coffee
- xylitol-sweetened soda or juice
- sparkling water
- xylitol
- vegetable juice
- dark chocolate with at least 70% cacao
- frozen plain bananas
- frozen plain berries

If You Fail to Plan, You Plan to Fail

Since low dopamine is associated with impulsivity, it's especially important for you to plan ahead. Have dopamine booster foods on hand when you come home in case you're in the habit of eating as soon as you walk in the door.

Dopamine Booster Activities

Through the twenty-eight days of Diet Rehab, you'll also be adding these booster activities to your daily life. Remember, you're the expert of you, and your feelings are information that indicates what you're needing at the moment. In the past, boredom would have mindlessly led you to a plate of chili cheese fries, but now you will be armed with a whole list of dopamine booster foods and activities you can use to fend off monotony.

Of course, have compassion toward yourself, and remember that low dopamine can be associated with hopelessness and sadness. So if this list of dopamine booster activities makes you feel overwhelmed, take a deep breath. Start slowly by adding five minutes of Sudoku and one dopamine booster snack to your mundane Monday. Or treat yourself to a game night to shake up your weekend routine. As your dopamine levels begin to climb, so will your motivation to tackle more and more on this list—and in your life. As you do, you'll probably discover some great dopamine booster activities of you own!

Act in community theater
Apply for a job
Ask a special someone on a date
Attend a 12-step meeting
Attend a lecture
Be the one to initiate sex tonight
Break down your list of goals into small, achievable subgoals
Browse property websites for a new house
Build something
Call in to a contest on a radio station
Clean the house to loud music and at a quick pace
Cook something you've never made before
Dance
Do a fast walk with your dog
Do some intense cardio or interval training
Do volunteer work that's rewarding and exciting
Drive a new way home from work
Dye your hair a new color . . . or let it go gray
Eat something you've never tried before

Fix something
Get a new haircut
Get eight hours of sleep
Get neurofeedback or EEG biofeedback
Get off at a train or bus stop in a part of town you've never been
    to before, or get in your car and drive to one
Get tickets to your favorite talk or game show
Get waxed
Go ballroom dancing
Go Kart
Go shark tank diving
Go to a 12-step meeting for the first time
Go to a bootcamp-style fitness class
Go to a city you've never been to before
Go to a restaurant you've never been to before
Go to a sporting event
Go to a zoo
Go to an open house just to look
Go to the target range
Go whitewater rafting
Go window shopping
Go wine tasting
Have a dance party with your kids
Have that conversation you've been meaning to have
Hike up a new trail
Hire a personal trainer
Hit some balls at a batting cage
Hit the playground with the kids
Host a theme party
Initiate foreplay
Invent something
Join a free meetup.com group—everything from hiking to groups
    just to meet new people

Join the PTA

Join Toastmasters, a public speaking group

Jump off the diving board into the pool

Jump rope

Karaoke

Kiss

Learn a new language

Learn how to salsa

Lift weights

Make a movie on your phone

Make an obstacle course for the kids—see who can do it the fastest

Make love

Make some really hot salsa

Meditate (download my dopamine booster meditation at www.drmikedow.com)

Miniature golf

Mountain bike

Order healthy takeout from a place you've never tried

Paint a room in your house a new color

Paint your nails a new color

Participate in a contest

Play a game or do a puzzle that challenges you, such as Sudoku, a crossword puzzle, a video game, poker

Play backgammon

Play ball

Play billiards

Play board games

Play bocce ball

Play darts

Play fetch with your dog

Play low-stakes poker with friends

Play Ping-Pong

Play soccer

Play tag

Play Twister

Poke around with one of those programs on your computer you've
never used before

Read an exhilarating novel or story

Read the comics

Read your horoscope

Rearrange your furniture

Ride a roller-coaster

Rollerblade

Sail

Scuba dive

See a therapist

Show up on time

Sign up for a dating website like match.com or eharmony.com

Sign up for speed dating

Ski

Snorkel

Snowmobile

Spend five minutes browsing vacation spots online

Sprint

Start a blog

Start a fantasy football league

Submit your short story to a magazine

Surprise your significant other with a romantic fantasy

Surprise your significant other with some sexy lingerie

Take a belly dancing or pole dancing class

Take a cold shower

Take a spin class

Take a trapeze lesson

Take a walk in the rain

Take part in a flash mob

Take the stairs
Take your dog to the dog park
Test drive a new car—buy it only if you can afford it
Text somebody and tell them why you appreciate them
Train for a 5K
Try a new sport, such as fencing, tennis, or surfing
Try on a new pair of shoes
Vote
Walk a new path
Watch a game show
Watch a horror or action movie
Watch a street performer
Watch airplanes take off
Watch competitive sports—better yet, play one
Wear a new color makeup today
Wear sexy underwear—even if it's just for you
Whiten your teeth
Write a song—and perform it for somebody
Write down five things you'd like to do this year
Write down ten things you'd like to do in your life

Dopamine Pitfall Foods

As you boost your dopamine with booster foods and activities, you'll be cutting back on the pitfalls listed below. The list I've provided isn't comprehensive, but it gives you a good indication of the kinds of things to avoid. When reading the nutrition label, be on the lookout for high levels of fat—especially saturated fat. When reading the ingredient list, too much oil and any partially hydrogenated oils can make some seemingly booster foods—like some "energy bars"—a pitfall food.

Remember, as your dopamine levels begin to rise, these former pitfalls will start to lose their seductive lure. But that doesn't mean they're not problematic and potentially addictive, so it's important to keep them at arm's length. Do a pitfall food raid in your kitchen as you begin to stock up on dopamine booster foods. Especially with the impulsivity associated with low dopamine, it's important to make sure these foods aren't easily accessible in moments of weakness or boredom. I want you to really think about what you want to eat before it goes in your mouth. That way, these pitfall foods will become occasional treats, not perennial parts of your everyday life.

Bacon
Breakfast pastries
Brownies
Spicy hot chicken wings
Butter
Cheese dip
Cookies
Corn chips
Cured meats like salami and Peperami
Deep-fried crackers
French fries
Fried foods
Full-fat coffee drinks
High-fat creamy cheese
Movie theater popcorn
Mozzarella sticks
Potato crisps
Sausage
Soda

By Leaps and Bounds

Whenever we focus on our strengths, we are setting ourselves up for success and happiness. Dopamine-craving types need novelty, adventure, and challenges. Now that you are armed with an arsenal of ways to get these needs met in healthy and sustainable ways, use that competitive streak in you to gradually yet powerfully commit to the life you know you want to live. It's not really about all the things you *can't* have; it's about getting what you really need so that the self-medicating substitutes fall by the wayside.

14

Diet Rehab: The Program

Now you're ready to start adding delicious booster foods and activities to your life! Here's the gradual detox program of Diet Rehab, which has you loading up on boosters and then—when you are starting to get what you need from your life—gradually cutting out pitfalls. To find suggestions of booster activities, see pages 208 and 223, and to find a list of booster foods, see pages 204 and 219.

As you already know, pitfall foods flood the brain with unsustainable amounts of serotonin and dopamine through saturated fats, sugars, and white carbohydrates. Yes, they are as bad for your brain as they are for your body!

Booster foods give your brain sustainable energy by promoting a healthy release of serotonin and dopamine, which is, of course, good for both brain and body. Thanks to the protein, healthy fats, and fiber they contain, booster foods also keep you feeling fuller for a longer period of time. Booster activities also promote healthy serotonin and dopamine levels, which will help you to decrease emotional eating and promote eating based on physical hunger. This combination of boosting will balance your brain chemistry, and, yes, you will actually begin to favor and even crave booster foods while feeling both physically and emotionally satisfied.

In weeks 1 and 2, you will add serotonin and/or dopamine booster foods, depending on which neurochemical you're really craving.

As your brain chemistry begins to become balanced in weeks 3 and 4, you can then fill your diet with any booster foods on pages 204 and 219. That means a person with low serotonin is free to try some dopamine booster foods, and those with low dopamine can add some serotonin booster foods. Our brains rely on healthy levels of both neurotransmitters to feel happy and healthy, and when you're feeling balanced and getting the excitement, happiness, or peace elsewhere, you will begin to benefit from any booster on these lists.

Armed with the knowledge of which boosters are particularly good for your brain chemistry, those low in serotonin can always favor serotonin booster foods. Also, you can favor them when you're feeling anxious or stressed out. Knowing that a whole apple with a cup of herbal tea is a serotonin booster food is a great weapon when you feel like you just can't handle one more thing at work, and it will also help you to bypass the vending machine candy bar.

Those low in dopamine can always favor dopamine booster foods. Reach for these foods when you're feeling low and need a pick-me-up. Knowing that plain, low-fat Greek yogurt with a cup of green tea is a dopamine booster food will help you pick yourself up when you're dragging, helping you to bypass the sugary energy drink and french fries.

Serotonin and dopamine booster foods have a lot more going for them than healthy levels of protein, good fats, and carbohydrates. They are also packed with one or more of the following healthy brain chemistry-promoting compounds: B-vitamins, amino acids, omega-3s, and protective antioxidants. For example, salmon—especially wild-caught—is a protein with fat, which means it helps to release dopamine, but it also contains so many brain-nourishing omega-3s that it's good for maintaining *both* serotonin and dopamine production. Blueberries—especially organic ones—have healthy levels of natural serotonin-boosting sugars, but they also have antioxidants that prevent damage to your neurons—helping them to continue pumping both serotonin and dopamine. Check out Appendix A for some of my favorite recipes using booster foods. These tools will help you make the booster food lists your grocery store list!

WEEK 1 = 1+1

- **Don't cut anything from your normal diet.** We add before we take away.
- **Make sure that at least ONE of your meals or snacks each day is made up of serotonin or dopamine booster foods.** See Part II to determine whether you are serotonin deficient, dopamine deficient, or both. If you need to replenish both types of brain chemical, alternate, adding a serotonin booster meal or snack one day and a dopamine booster meal or snack the next.
- **Add ONE booster activity each day.** Based on your findings in Part II as to whether you are serotonin deficient, dopamine deficient, or both, booster activities will replenish the neurochemicals you need most. If you need to replenish both serotonin and dopamine, alternate, adding a serotonin booster one day and a dopamine booster the next.

WEEK 2 = 2+2

- **Don't cut anything from your normal diet.**
- **Make sure that at least TWO of your meals or snacks each day are made up of serotonin or dopamine booster foods.** If you need to replenish both types of brain chemical, add one serotonin and one dopamine booster meal or snack each day.
- **Add TWO serotonin or dopamine booster activities each day.**

WEEK 3 = 3-3

• Limit your pitfall foods to no more than THREE servings per day. The rest of all meals and snacks will be made up of booster foods. Favor boosters tailored to your brain chemistry, but now that your brain chemistry is beginning to be balanced, any booster food will start to be beneficial. A pitfall food serving is around 300 calories at most, so you're going for a maximum of about 900 calories from pitfall foods.

• Add THREE serotonin or dopamine booster activities each day. See Part II to determine whether you are serotonin deficient, dopamine deficient, or both. If you need to replenish both types of brain chemical, alternate between adding two serotonin boosters and one dopamine booster and adding one serotonin booster and two dopamine boosters.

WEEK 4 = 4-2

• Limit your pitfall foods to no more than TWO servings per day. Everything else you eat should be boosters. Favor boosters tailored to your brain chemistry, but now that your brain chemistry is beginning to be balanced, any booster food will start to be beneficial. Remember, one serving of a pitfall food is about 300 calories, so you're looking at a maximum of about 600 calories of pitfall foods.

• Add FOUR serotonin or dopamine booster activities each day. See Part II to determine whether you are serotonin deficient, dopamine deficient, or both. If you need to replenish both types of brain chemical, add two boosters of each type every day.

MAINTENANCE = 4-2

• Limit your pitfall foods to no more than TWO servings per day. The rest of all meals and snacks will be made up of boosters. Favor boosters tailored to your brain chemistry, but now that your brain chemistry is beginning to be balanced, any booster food will start to be beneficial. Remember, one serving of a pitfall food is about 300 calories, so you're looking at a maximum of about 600 calories of pitfall foods.

- **Maintain FOUR booster activities each day.** Favor booster activities tailored to your brain chemistry (low serotonin or low dopamine), but now that your brain chemistry is beginning to be balanced, any booster activity will start to be beneficial. Low serotonin types may want to add a few dopamine booster activities, especially when they feel like they need an energizing lift. Low dopamine types may want to add a few serotonin booster activities, especially when they need some peace and calm. Dual-deficiency types can continue to add from both dopamine booster and serotonin booster activities lists.

Journal Your Way to Weight Loss

One of the simplest and clinically most effective ways to lose weight is to keep a food journal. You will be adding accountability to each meal and snack by writing down everything you consume, helping you to become more mindful and less likely to choose impulsively.

The Diet Rehab journal has some other key elements. First, you will be tracking booster activities in addition to your food. You will also be writing about the way your daily efforts to balance your brain chemicals positively affects your mantra and your mood. This improvement in the way you feel is the ultimate reward, and this positive feedback will help you to keep your life going in the upward spiral you've created. If you've felt that your mood is entirely out of your control, writing about your activities and their results will give you a sense of hope, as most of your mood is actually in your control, based on your daily choices to take care of your health, your body, and your life.

Join Our Online Community!

Knowing you're not alone and getting support from others can help you keep going and also turn struggles into triumphs. That's why I created the Diet Rehab Community on my website, www.drmikedow.com. Visit the site to post some of your favorite booster food recipes or to read some from other members of our community. Share your experience, hear stories of hope, and get tips from others who know what you're going through. Visit www.drmikedow.com, and get connected!

The Diet Rehab Plan: Frequently Asked Questions

Q. What if I really love pasta?
A. No problem! Just make it the old-school Italian way, where at least 20 to 30 percent of the pasta dish is actually booster foods like tomatoes, artichokes, garlic, and herbs with a sprinkling of extra-virgin olive oil. Add a salad or a portion of green vegetables that is as big as the pasta dish to really maximize the satiety of the meal. And swap your white-flour pasta for boosting whole-wheat or high-protein pasta. If you're stuck somewhere eating the pitfall version of this food, just count each serving as one of your pitfall servings for that day.

Q. Which vegetables are pitfalls and which are boosters?
A. Potatoes give you a quick, addictive rush of serotonin, so they are the only vegetable classified as a pitfall food. All other vegetables—including sweet potatoes—give your brain a healthy, sustainable dose of serotonin, so they are all booster foods. Vegetables also have a high-satiety value, so they'll help you feel full. Make sure you're opting for

veggies that aren't fried or cooked in a lot of butter or oil. A deep-fried vegetable counts as a pitfall food.

Q. Which fruits are pitfalls and which are boosters?
A. Any fruit that has not been tampered with is a booster, except for serotonin-spiking dates, pineapples, or watermelon. All other fruits may be fresh, cut, or frozen. They must not have added sugar, oil, syrup, not be juiced, not preserved, not dried, and not canned. I keep frozen organic blueberries and raspberries (with no added sugar) in my freezer at all times, as they are a fantastic addition to oatmeal and my favorite nonfat Greek yogurt. As an added bonus, the skins of apples, pears, plums, and peaches are high in fiber and therefore high on the satiety index.

Q. What if I don't have time to cook?
A. I know what you mean—I don't either! Check out my favorite booster food recipes in Appendix A, where I share a week's worth of meals that take less than twenty minutes to prepare.

Q. Shouldn't I be exercising, too?
A. Our bodies were made to move, and I'd like you to exercise yours. But unless you're already engaged in a satisfying exercise program, I'm suggesting you start slow, because you are just beginning to heal your brain chemistry—which is why you add only one booster activity in week 1 and then four per day by week 4. You'll notice that many of the booster activities on pages 208 and 223 are physical, and as you start to feel better, it will become easier and easier to add more forms of booster exercise to your day.

Q. Do I have to give up drinking?
A. If you have a problem with alcohol, you must first seek the advice of your physician before beginning this program. Diet Rehab is not de-

signed to treat alcoholism. Otherwise, I encourage everyone to limit their daily alcohol intake, to about one serving for non-alcoholic women and two for non-alcoholic men. At these numbers, you are reducing your risk of many major diseases. Anything more than this and you will actually increase your risk of many major diseases, not to mention putting you at risk for alcoholism. Alcohol contains a huge amount of calories (big frozen drinks can sometimes pack about 500), and drinking lowers your inhibitions around food, making you more likely to snack when you're not hungry. Of course, count all sugary mixers such as tonic water or juice as a serving of pitfall food.

Ever notice how you crave salty, fatty snacks when you have a drink? Alcohol is also a pitfall in that it overstimulates your brain chemistry, leaving you in a slump the next day, leading you to consume more pitfall foods in an attempt to soothe your frazzled nerves and lift yourself out of depression.

In general, I advise my patients not to drink their calories. It's not satisfying to drink a milk shake and be told you just had a whole day's intake of fat, or to overdo the wine drinking and realize you just took two steps back on your feeling-good mission.

Q. I'm never going to give up red meat.
A: And you don't have to! You can find cuts of beef that are at least 95% lean. You can also always have that burger or hot dog at the baseball game that are more than 5% fat. Just count that small burger or hot dog as one serving of a pitfall food.

Q. I'm on a special diet: diabetic, gluten-free, kosher, for food allergies, vegetarian, vegan . . .
A: No worries. You may have to choose from a somewhat more restricted list of choices, but you can definitely find booster foods that will fit the limits you're working within.

Q. *What about salad dressings?*
A: I recommend a teaspoon of healthy extra-virgin olive oil (a fantastic booster food) mixed with as much vinegar (I recommend balsamic, white, red, cider, or champagne vinegars) or lemon juice as you like. Remember that most store-bought and restaurant dressings contain huge amounts of sugar and unhealthy fats.

Q. *Why don't I have to think about calories?*
A: Lean proteins, non-starchy vegetables, and whole fruits have fewer calories per ounce than starches or fatty meats. If you focus on consuming lots of boosters, you'll fill up on healthy food that supports your brain chemistry and satisfies your hunger and you'll automatically and naturally be consuming fewer calories. The amount of food you will take in will begin to self-regulate once you are feeling better and have let go of your food addictions. Our bodies were meant to be hungry for the amount of calories they need. We just need to start listening to that physical hunger.

Q. *What about diet soda and juice?*
A: Vegetable juice is great since it has a fraction of the serotonin-spiking sugar that fruit juice has, so it's a booster food. Juice—even all-natural fruit juice—has a high concentration of sugar, which floods your brain with serotonin the same way sugar in soda can. As for diet soda, it may not have calories, but it does calibrate your taste buds to a super-sweet level that leads you to shun natural sweetness and causes you to crave sweet, starchy foods. If you need a replacement to wean yourself off diet soda, look for xylitol-sweetened sodas. Better yet, choose flavored sparkling waters, flavored teas, or coffee. Count fruit juice, soda, and diet soda as pitfall foods. The only exception to this are xylitol-sweetened fruit juices and sodas which count as booster foods.

Q. What about artificial sweeteners?

A: There is only one artificial sweetener classified as a booster food: xylitol. Hopefully you will use this only occasionally because you'll become more tolerant of the natural sweetness of whole foods. If you are a honey, maple syrup, or preserves person, there are some xylitol-based varieties of all three. Let them be a little treat, as too much can also cause digestive problems. If you are a need-five-Splenda-in-my-coffee person, as I used to be, xylitol is a great option: it's not as sweet as other artificial sweeteners, and it will help you to recalibrate your taste buds baby step by baby step. Hopefully you will eventually like your coffee black or with just a splash of skim milk like I do now. And when you are looking for something sweet, you can go right to the grocery store and load up on all your favorite booster fruits.

Q. What about sugar-free gum?

A: When it comes to choosing anything in our lives, we always have to consider if the benefit outweighs the risk. The amount of artificial sweetener in sugar-free gum is negligible, and it's great for preventing cavities and keeping your breath fresh!

Q. What if I mess up and don't have enough booster foods or booster activities, or have too many pitfalls in one day?

A: You now know that polarized thinking is a pitfall. That means that if you have one day where you mess up, it does *not* mean that your *whole* Diet Rehab is now ruined. Nor should you engage in personalization, another pitfall style of thinking, where one bad day means that *you* are just too weak or a failure.

What you should do is simply move on to the next day. Now maybe you think that you should punish yourself. Perhaps you think if you had four pitfall food servings on day twenty-four when you were supposed to have only two, having *no* pitfall foods on day twenty-five is a great way to make up for this.

This cycle of punishment actually makes things worse. One extreme type of food addiction is binge-eating disorder. When a binge eater has binged, the most clinically effective way to deal with the next meal or snack is to eat *as if the binge hadn't happened*. That's right: Even if a binge eater had 2,000 calories at four a.m., he or she will actually benefit from going ahead and eating a normal breakfast as opposed to skipping the next two meals to compensate for the binge. The same principle applies to all eaters. When you start punishing yourself by compensating, you are affirming a mantra of "I'm bad and need to be punished." In the long run, this actually sets you up for failure and not success. Just keep following the plan day by day, no matter what you did the day before.

Q. *What if I relapse after my 28-day Diet Rehab?*
A. You may find yourself sneaking three pitfall foods back into your diet, and the following month, you're back up to four. Now that you know how food is addictive, you will realize that this puts you back in danger of needing more and more fatty and sugary food just to feel normal.

Relapse is especially common when you have something difficult or stressful in your life. Use the unexpected tragedies, obstacles, and transitions in your life as an opportunity to be even more diligent in getting what you need through booster foods and activities that will help you to take care of yourself. It's normal to experience sadness and anxiety when going through difficult life incidents, and we all want to feel better when this happens. The only question is: Will you choose unhealthy self-medication through pitfall foods, or will you find healthier ways to take care of your feelings through booster foods and activities?

Don't be hard on yourself. Just use every relapse as an opportunity that tells you there's still something in your life you are not getting enough of. Perhaps the first time around you felt happier but you still weren't getting the support you needed. Maybe the second time around you can decide to start psychotherapy, hire a trainer, or go to an Overeaters Anonymous meeting in addition to all of the other healthy rituals that are now a part of your life. If you're still feeling out of control, then perhaps that feeling is telling you it's time to consider an inpatient or an intensive outpatient program to treat your food and weight issues; you can go to www.drmikedow.com for referrals and my help line.

If Someone You Love Is a Food Addict . . .

Remember that food addicts get so much negative feedback already in the form of judgment and criticism from themselves and others. What they need is your love and support. The best way to display this is to model healthy behavior and nonverbally show your support by doing things like cooking a healthy meal or taking a walk with him or her. Don't make them feel alienated by cooking a "special" meal for them unless they have asked for it. You will help the whole family by cooking with booster foods that are good for everyone's health.

When talking to your loved one, move from "you" language to "I" language. So instead of "You really need to lose weight. Are you sure you want to eat that?" say, "I feel really worried about your health. I love you and want to support you. Is there anything I can do?"

Don't enable a food addict by buying pitfall foods at the grocery store. But it's not your responsibility to police them by watching over every bite either. Somewhere in the middle of enabling and policing is supporting, and that's where you want to be to help a food addict. Remember, the decision to change must ultimately come from them.

Interventions aren't just for drug addicts and alcoholics. If someone you love is a true food addict and you don't know what else to do, a professionally moderated food intervention can be an effective way to promote healthy family communication and get the addict the help he or she needs. Go to www.drmikedow.com for more information about food interventions and referrals for inpatient and intensive outpatient programs for food addicts.

Booster Snacks and Meals

Trying to figure out how to incorporate booster foods into your diet?
Here are some suggestions:

SEROTONIN BOOSTER SNACKS	SEROTONIN BOOSTER MEALS
• 1 cup cottage cheese with ½ cup berries • 2 squares of dark chocolate and herbal tea • Whole-wheat tortilla with hummus and 1 apple, sparkling water • Carrot and beet juice and light CheeseString • Banana, 1 cup plain Greek yogurt, flavored tea • Carrots and hummus, sparkling water • Whole-wheat English muffin with fat-free cream cheese, hot water with lemon	• Whole-wheat pasta, marinara sauce with broccoli, ½ cup berries with xylitol • Turkey on whole-wheat bread with light Swiss cheese, 1 apple, white tea • Large beet and leafy green salad with low-fat Italian dressing with grilled salmon, 1 whole-wheat roll, decaf coffee • ½ cup cooked brown rice, grilled mahi-mahi, sautéed red and yellow peppers, ¼ cup blueberries, and 1 cup plain Greek yogurt • Grilled chicken strips over leafy greens, ¼ cup low-fat cheddar cheese, salsa, 1 piece of whole-wheat toast

DOPAMINE BOOSTER SNACKS	DOPAMINE BOOSTER MEALS
• 1 cup plain Greek yogurt, small black coffee • Light string cheese, 1 whole apple, large green tea • Carrots with hummus, vegetable juice, sparkling water • Egg white wrap in whole-wheat tortilla and light feta cheese • 6 slices of low-sodium deli turkey, 1 whole apple • 10 almonds, light CheeseString, sparkling water • Small decaf with ¼ cup skim milk and 2 hard-boiled eggs • 8 celery sticks and salsa, coffee with a splash of skim milk • 2 cups reduced-fat microwaved popcorn, 1 whole peach	• 2 grilled chicken breasts, grilled broccoli, plain Greek yogurt with frozen blueberries • Turkey chili, romaine lettuce salad with balsamic vinegar and olive oil, 1 whole pear • 4 ounces grilled wild salmon, side of spinach sautéed in olive oil and garlic, 1 cup of skim milk • Grilled grass-fed 95% lean beef patty, 1 slice of low-fat Swiss cheese on a bed of mixed leafy greens topped with avocado, spicy mustard, and balsamic vinegar

Keep Your Pitfalls Manageable

As you choose pitfall foods, be sure that you're choosing manageable servings that won't flood your brain with chemicals and restart your addictions. If there is something not on this list or if you're not sure what one serving means, then remember that a pitfall-food serving contains no more than about 300 calories.

1 MANAGEABLE SERVING OF PITFALL FOOD:

- 12 ounces of fruit juice
- 2 sausage links
- 1 small pancake
- 2 tablespoons maple syrup or artificially flavored syrup
- 1 bagel
- 2 tablespoons full-fat cream cheese
- 1 small doughnut
- 1 piece of coffee cake
- 1 cup whole milk
- Home fries
- 1 croissant
- 1 small muffin
- 1 piece of full-fat cheese
- 1 biscuit
- 1 slice of pepperoni pizza
- 6 ounces flavored full-sugar yogurt
- 1 piece of fried chicken
- 3 chicken nuggets
- 4-ounce serving of red meat containing more than 5% fat
- Small coleslaw
- Small french fries
- 1 serving of mashed potatoes
- 1 baked potato
- 1 hot dog
- 1 serving of baked beans
- 2 tablespoons peanut butter

1 MANAGEABLE SERVING OF PITFALL FOOD:

- 2 tablespoons of jelly or jam
- 2 ounces of white pasta
- Alfredo or cheese sauce
- 2 meatballs
- Small cheeseburger
- Tuna or chicken salad in full-fat mayonnaise
- 2 pieces white bread
- Large flour tortilla
- 12 saltines or crackers
- Small bag of crisps
- Nuts roasted in oil
- Dried fruit in oil
- Fruit cocktail in syrup
- Small bag of pretzels
- ½ of a small movie theater popcorn
- ½ of a small order of nachos
- ½ of a large pretzel
- Side of cheese sauce
- Ramen noodles
- ⅓ box of macaroni and cheese
- 8-ounce milk shake
- 1 slice of cheesecake
- 1 piece of cake
- 1 cup frozen yogurt
- 1 cup ice cream
- 12 ounces soda
- 12 ounces diet soda
- 12 ounces tonic water
- 1 small iced sugary coffee beverage
- 12 ounces fruit juice
- 2 small cookies
- Small candy bar
- Small milk chocolate bar
- 6 pieces of licorice
- 2 tablespoons full-fat salad dressing

1 MANAGEABLE SERVING OF PITFALL FOOD:
• 2 tablespoons full-fat mayonnaise
• 2 tablespoons tartar sauce
• 1 tablespoon butter, margarine, or oil (except olive oil)
• 2 tablespoons sugar

Swaps and Switches

One of the most exciting aspects of rehabbing your diet from the perpetual frustration of yo-yo dieting is the way Diet Rehab focuses on what you're adding, not on what you're taking away. You're always going to like certain foods, such as pasta or orange juice. But with a few simple tweaks, you can get the taste you're craving in a more healthy and sustainable way. As you follow this program, you will actually begin to prefer these booster foods over the pitfall foods they're replacing! I know from my own personal experience. But don't take my word for it. Experience it for yourself.

INSTEAD OF THIS PITFALL	SWAP WITH THIS BOOSTER FOOD
• coffee with sugar	• flavored-bean coffee
• orange juice	• whole orange
• apple juice	• whole apple
• bacon	• turkey bacon
• fruit-on-the-bottom yogurt	• plain yogurt with xylitol and frozen blueberries
• banana-flavored oatmeal	• plain oatmeal with ½ banana
• white bread	• whole-wheat bread (3 or more grams of fiber)
• cream cheese	• fat-free cream cheese
• corn flakes or puffed rice cereal	• whole-wheat cereal (5 or more grams of fiber)
• cranberry juice cocktail	• sparkling water
• soda	• coffee or tea
• tonic water	• soda water

INSTEAD OF THIS PITFALL	SWAP WITH THIS BOOSTER FOOD
• Caesar dressing	• vinaigrette
• ranch dressing	• balsamic vinegar
• Thousand Island dressing	• lemon and pepper
• croutons	• whole-wheat bread (more than 3 grams fiber)
• half-and-half	• skim milk
• non-dairy creamer	• 1% milk
• small cheeseburger	• 3-ounce sirloin steak (less than 5% fat)
• burger on white bun	• veggie burger, whole-wheat bun
• french fries	• baked sweet potato
• orange chicken	• Szechuan chicken
• saag paneer (spinach and cheese)	• bhindi bhajee (okra in tomato sauce)
• egg roll	• grilled chicken skewers
• spicy tuna roll wrapped with white rice	• tuna sashimi, side of edamame
• 1 cup of white rice	• ½ cup of brown rice and extra steamed vegetables
• 6-inch cold-cut submarine sandwich on white bread with American cheese, mayonnaise, and salt and pepper, crisps soda	• 6-inch turkey submarine sandwich on wheat bread, no cheese, extra vegetables, extra vinegar, mustard, black pepper, side of cut apples, decaf coffee
• BK Whopper, large onion rings, soda	• BK veggie burger patty put on top of salad, reduced-fat Italian dressing, water
• Big Mac, large fries, chocolate milk shake	• Grilled chicken salad, vinaigrette, water
• guacamole	• extra salsa
• Spanish rice	• extra grilled bell peppers
• beef fajitas in flour tortillas	• grilled shrimp fajitas, no tortillas
• flour tortilla	• whole-wheat tortilla
• sour cream	• Tabasco
• fried chicken	• grilled chicken
• cheese sauce	• hummus
• peanut butter	• almond butter
• cream-based soup	• broth-based soup
• lots of noodles	• lots of vegetables
• beef chili	• turkey or veggie chili
• ranch dip	• salsa
• potato crisps	• soy crisps

247

INSTEAD OF THIS PITFALL	SWAP WITH THIS BOOSTER FOOD
• cheddar cheese	• light cheese
• white pasta	• whole-wheat pasta
• salt	• black pepper
• mayo	• reduced-fat mayo
• butter	• 1 tablespoon olive oil
• oil	• mustard
• candy bar	• protein bar (more than 15 grams protein)
• saltines with peanut butter	• carrots or celery with hummus or salsa
• crisps	• whole apple
• milk chocolate	• 70% or more cacao chocolate
• apple pie	• frozen whole banana
• chocolate milk shake	• chocolate whey shake
• fruit pastry	• granola bar (more than 5 grams fiber)
• frozen yogurt with strawberries in syrup	• plain low-fat Greek yogurt with frozen whole strawberries, xylitol
• fried	• baked, sautéed, grilled
• heavy-handed oil (even olive oil)	• light-handed oil, heavy-handed vinegar and spices
• visible fat present	• trim it
• visible grease present	• blot it

Beware the Stealth Foods

Finally, beware the pitfall foods in disguise—foods that appear healthy but are really loaded with sugar, starch, fat, or salt. Check out the following list:

PITFALL FOODS IN DISGUISE
• protein or energy bars with less than 15 grams of protein
• breakfast, fiber, or granola bars with less than 5 grams of fiber
• dark chocolate with less than 70% cacao
• wheat bread with less than 3 grams of fiber per serving

PITFALL FOODS IN DISGUISE
• dried fruit made with oil
• sugary sodas that market themselves as "naturally flavored"
• fruit juice
• frozen yogurt
• frozen fruit toppings in sugar
• "real fruit" smoothies that use fruits in sugar or juice
• anything with high-fructose corn syrup
• anything with partially hydrogenated oils or trans fats

Set Yourself Up for Success

Choosing to commit to something *when you're ready* ensures that this change is coming from the most important place: you. The best predictor for success is your *willingness* to change. When you are truly ready to make a change in your life, then it's time to manifest the health and happiness you've been longing for.

Goals that are made in public are more likely to be kept than goals made in private. So it's time to go beyond the resolutions you make to yourself in your head—the same resolutions that aren't likely to be kept. Make your journey public. Tell your significant other, friend, 12-step sponsor, trainer, or health care professional, and have them sign this contract with you. You'll be making a binding promise to the most important person in this agreement—you—and it's a simple way to keep yourself accountable and get the support you will need on this journey.

Here's your Diet Rehab contract:

I've identified that my pitfall mantra is: _____

_____

And the mantra that I'd like to have is: _____

_____

The best thing about having this new mantra will be: _____

_____

I would rate my willingness to make a change on a scale of 0 to 10 (with 0 being not willing to lift a finger and 10 being willing to do whatever it takes): _____

My current weight: _____

My goal weight: _____
(Set yourself an achievable weight-loss goal for the 28-day period of Diet Rehab. This might be anything from two to ten pounds. Remember, setting achievable goals is one of the ways to avoid pitfall styles of thinking.)

I, *(your name)* _____, am committed to following Diet Rehab for *twenty-eight* days. I will eat booster foods and fill my life with booster activities that will change my mantra. I will actively change any obsessive, emotional, or compulsive eating using the tools I now have. Embarking on this journey means that I am affirming my own self-worth, and I am willing to let my behaviors and choices help support this belief.

Signed,   Date:

_____   _____

(You)

_____   _____

(Accountability buddy: friend, spouse, health care professional, sponsor)

Below you'll find a sample serotonin deficient, dopamine deficient, and dual deficiency food journal for each week.

Serotonin-Deficient Food Journal

Circle your serotonin booster meal or snack (they are in italics and boldface).

Breakfast: sugary cereal with milk, croissant, orange juice, coffee with sugar and cream

Lunch: 2 pieces of garlic bread, spaghetti in marinara sauce, 2 sodas

Dinner: *dinner salad made with romaine lettuce, tomatoes in balsamic vinaigrette, 1 cup of brown rice, 1 breast of grilled chicken with fresh rosemary, thyme, and black pepper, 2 glasses of sparkling water*

Snack (optional): king-size candy bar, soda

Snack (optional): crisps, water

Snack (optional): 2 cups of chocolate ice cream

Booster activity: took a 10-minute walk in the afternoon when I was feeling stressed

Serotonin-Deficient Food Journal

Circle your serotonin booster meals or snacks (they are in italics and boldface).

Breakfast: whole milk latte, muffin

Lunch: *brown rice bowl with sliced steamed carrots, broccoli, and grilled black sole with low-sodium soy sauce, green tea*

Dinner: club sandwich, fries, sweetened iced tea

Snack (optional): candy

Snack (optional): *protein bar, decaf coffee with skim milk*

Snack (optional): pretzels

Booster activity 1: meditated for five minutes in the morning

Booster activity 2: challenged myself by saying hello to a stranger in the elevator when I was going to work

Serotonin-Deficient Food Journal

Circle your maximum of 3 servings of pitfall foods (they are in italics and boldface).

Breakfast: whole pear, instant oatmeal with xylitol, hot white tea

Lunch: *2 pieces of pepperoni pizza (2),* green salad with low-fat Italian dressing, water

Dinner: high-fiber pasta with marinara sauce, grilled chicken, and red bell peppers, sparkling water

Snack (optional): baby carrots with hummus, hot water with lemon

Snack (optional): *small bag of crisps (1)*

Snack (optional): none

Booster activity 1: sent a nice e-mail telling a friend how much I appreciate him

Booster activity 2: prayed and gave thanks for things I was grateful for today

Booster activity 3: took a nap in the sun for twenty minutes

Serotonin-Deficient Food Journal

Circle your maximum of 2 servings of pitfall foods (they are in italics and boldface).

Breakfast: high-fiber granola bar, whole orange, green tea

Lunch: grilled chicken Caesar salad, no croutons, with low-fat dressing, sparkling water

Dinner: grilled tilapia, steamed green beans, ½ cup brown rice

Snack (optional): *dried fruit snacks (1)*

Snack (optional): bowl of low-sodium vegetable soup

Snack (optional): *small bag of crisps (1)*

Booster activity 1: cuddled with my dog for ten minutes before work

Booster activity 2: cleaned my closet

Booster activity 3: took a thirty-minute walk after dinner

Booster activity 4: went to my ceramics class

Dopamine-Deficient Food Journal

Circle your dopamine booster meal or snack (they are in italics and boldface).

Breakfast: sausage, white toast with peanut butter, orange juice, 2 cups of coffee with nondairy creamer

Lunch: cheeseburger, fries, diet soda

Dinner: *high-protein pasta with grilled shrimp, asparagus, and broccoli in marinara sauce, green tea, fat-free Greek yogurt with organic frozen blueberries*

Snack (optional): crisps, diet soda

Snack (optional): milk chocolate

Snack (optional): chocolate muffin

Booster activity: lifted weights for forty minutes

Dopamine-Deficient Food Journal

Circle your dopamine booster meals or snacks (they are in italics and boldface).

Breakfast: *low-fat plain Greek yogurt with frozen raspberries, coffee with low-fat milk*

Lunch: shrimp fried rice, 2 egg rolls, white rice with soy sauce, soda

Dinner: fried chicken, biscuits with gravy, corn on the cob with butter, water

Snack (optional): *protein bar*

Snack (optional): 2 candy bars

Snack (optional): large bag of crisps, frozen coffee beverage with whole milk, sugar

Booster activity 1: went to an Overeaters Anonymous meeting for the first time

Booster activity 2: played fetch with my dog for twenty minutes

Dopamine-Deficient Food Journal

Circle your maximum of 3 servings of pitfall foods (they are in italics and boldface).

Breakfast: whey protein powder mixed with skim milk, banana, frozen mixed berries

Lunch: grilled mahimahi on a bed of mixed greens, tomatoes, walnuts in balsamic vinegar and olive oil

Dinner: *small cheeseburger (1), small french fries (1)*, bottle of water

Snack (optional): fried chicken snack wrap (1)

Snack (optional): low-fat cheese, ten plain almonds, black coffee

Snack (optional): *small soda (1)*, whole apple

Booster activity 1: watched my favorite sports team for thirty minutes

Booster activity 2: took a walk around my neighborhood and followed a new route

Booster activity 3: looked at vacation spots online

Dopamine-Deficient Food Journal

Circle your maximum of 2 servings of pitfall foods (they are in italics and boldface).

Breakfast: *breakfast pastry (1)*, black coffee

Lunch: veggie burger with spicy mustard on whole-wheat bun, baked sweet potato fries, large unsweetened iced coffee

Dinner: high-protein pasta with grilled chicken breast and rosemary in a spicy marinara sauce, whole-wheat garlic bread made with lots of fresh garlic and a little extra-virgin olive oil

Snack (optional): hard-boiled egg, green tea

Snack (optional): *small cheeseburger (1)*

Snack (optional): ten almonds, ½ cup fresh blueberries

Booster activity 1: spin class

Booster activity 2: drove home a new way from work

Booster activity 3: bought flowers for my wife

Booster activity 4: made love

Dual-Deficiency Food Journal

Circle your serotonin or dopamine booster meal or snack (they are in italics and boldface).

Breakfast: 2 toaster pastries, orange juice

Lunch: *grilled salmon in olive oil and black pepper, ½ cup quinoa, steamed broccoli, coffee with a splash of skim milk, water*

Dinner: steak, baked potato, corn in butter sauce, water

Snack (optional): ten saltines, diet soda

Snack (optional): small bag of crisps

Snack (optional): carrot juice, whole apple, ten almonds

Booster activity: called a friend I haven't talked to in a long time

Dual-Deficiency Food Journal

Circle your serotonin and dopamine booster meals or snacks (they are in italics and boldface).

Breakfast: *Kashi high-fiber cereal, skim milk, frozen mixed berries, ½ banana, hot black tea*

Lunch: cold-cut sub, crisps, diet soda

Dinner: pasta in cream sauce, garlic bread, beer

Snack (optional): *whole apple, low-fat CheeseString*

Snack (optional): crackers

Snack (optional): croissant

Booster activity 1: wrote in my journal

Booster activity 2: signed up for Meals On Wheels training

Dual-Deficiency Food Journal

Circle your maximum of 3 servings of pitfall foods (they are in italics and boldface).

Breakfast: *hash browns (1)*, scrambled eggs, coffee with xylitol, water

Lunch: tuna salad with reduced-fat mayo, lettuce, tomato on whole-wheat bread, whole apple, unsweetened iced tea

Dinner: grilled chicken, low-fat cheese, salsa, fat-free sour cream in a whole-wheat tortilla, celery with salsa, water

Snack (optional): Vitamin Water Zero, whole apple, ten almonds

Snack (optional): *small candy bar (1)*

Snack (optional): *2 pieces of white bread (1)*, 2 tablespoons almond butter

Booster activity 1: saw my therapist

Booster activity 2: went to bed thirty minutes earlier to feel well rested tomorrow

Booster activity 3: took the stairs instead of the elevator at work

Dual-Deficiency Food Journal

Circle your maximum of 2 servings of pitfall foods (they are in italics and boldface).

Breakfast: whole grapefruit, low-fat CheeseString, green tea, water

Lunch: *2 pieces of white bread (1)*, filet mignon, steamed broccoli, *french fries (1)*

Dinner: quinoa in balsamic vinegar and extra-virgin olive oil, grilled salmon, mixed grilled vegetables in light pesto glaze

Snack (optional): protein bar

Snack (optional): celery with salsa

Snack (optional): whole apple, light CheeseString

Booster activity 1: played ball with my son outside for forty-five minutes

Booster activity 2: did a favor for my neighbor when I picked up her son from school

Booster activity 3: ate at a new restaurant

Booster activity 4: sent a thank-you card to a friend

Here's where you can journal your own Diet Rehab progress:

Day 1, Week 1

Circle your booster meal or snack.

Breakfast _____
_____

Lunch _____
_____

Dinner _____
_____

Snack (optional) _____
Snack (optional) _____
Snack (optional) _____

Booster activity _____
_____

Day 2, Week 1

Circle your booster meal or snack.

Breakfast _____

_____

Lunch _____

_____

Dinner _____

_____

Snack (optional) _____

Snack (optional) _____

Snack (optional) _____

Booster activity _____

_____

Day 3, Week 1

Circle your booster meal or snack.

Breakfast _____
_____

Lunch _____
_____

Dinner _____
_____

Snack (optional) _____
Snack (optional) _____
Snack (optional) _____

Booster activity _____
_____

Day 4, Week 1

Circle your booster meal or snack.

Breakfast _____

_____

Lunch _____

_____

Dinner _____

_____

Snack (optional) _____

Snack (optional) _____

Snack (optional) _____

Booster activity _____

_____

Day 5, Week 1

Circle your booster meal or snack.

Breakfast _____
_____

Lunch _____
_____

Dinner _____
_____

Snack (optional) _____
Snack (optional) _____
Snack (optional) _____

Booster activity _____
_____

Day 6, Week 1

Circle your booster meal or snack.

Breakfast _____

_____

Lunch _____

_____

Dinner _____

_____

Snack (optional) _____

Snack (optional) _____

Snack (optional) _____

Booster activity _____

_____

Day 7, Week 1

Circle your booster meal or snack.

Breakfast _____

_____

Lunch _____

_____

Dinner _____

_____

Snack (optional) _____

Snack (optional) _____

Snack (optional) _____

Booster activity _____

_____

My weight: _____ **pounds**

What I learned about myself this week was: _____
_____
_____

What I think I need more of in my life is: _____
_____
_____

The thing I'm most proud of myself this week is: _____
_____
_____

I have noticed the seven pitfall thought patterns (personalization, pervasiveness, paralysis-analysis, pessimism, polarization, psychic, permanence):

INCREASED   DECREASED   REMAINED THE SAME

I have felt the seven booster attributes (purpose, peace, pride, power, passion, productivity, pleasure) in my life:

INCREASED   DECREASED   REMAINED THE SAME

Overall, I'm feeling: _____
_____
_____

Day 8, Week 2

Circle your 2 booster meals or snacks.

Breakfast _____

_____

Lunch _____

_____

Dinner _____

_____

Snack (optional) _____

Snack (optional) _____

Snack (optional) _____

Booster activity 1 _____

_____

Booster activity 2 _____

_____

Day 9, Week 2

Circle your 2 booster meals or snacks.

Breakfast _____

_____

Lunch _____

_____

Dinner _____

_____

Snack (optional) _____

Snack (optional) _____

Snack (optional) _____

Booster activity 1 _____

_____

Booster activity 2 _____

_____

Day 10, Week 2

Circle your 2 booster meals or snacks.

Breakfast _____

_____

Lunch _____

_____

Dinner _____

_____

Snack (optional) _____

Snack (optional) _____

Snack (optional) _____

Booster activity 1 _____

_____

Booster activity 2 _____

_____

Day 11, Week 2

Circle your 2 booster meals or snacks.

Breakfast _____

_____

Lunch _____

_____

Dinner _____

_____

Snack (optional) _____

Snack (optional) _____

Snack (optional) _____

Booster activity 1 _____

_____

Booster activity 2 _____

_____

Day 12, Week 2

Circle your 2 booster meals or snacks.

Breakfast _____

_____

Lunch _____

_____

Dinner _____

_____

Snack (optional) _____

Snack (optional) _____

Snack (optional) _____

Booster activity 1 _____

_____

Booster activity 2 _____

_____

Day 13, Week 2

Circle your 2 booster meals or snacks.

Breakfast _____

_____

Lunch _____

_____

Dinner _____

_____

Snack (optional) _____

Snack (optional) _____

Snack (optional) _____

Booster activity 1 _____

_____

Booster activity 2 _____

_____

Day 14, Week 2

Circle your 2 booster meals or snacks.

Breakfast _____
_____

Lunch _____
_____

Dinner _____
_____

Snack (optional) _____
Snack (optional) _____
Snack (optional) _____

Booster activity 1 _____
_____

Booster activity 2 _____
_____

My weight: _____ **pounds**

What I learned about myself this week was: _____
_____
_____

What I think I need more of in my life is: _____
_____
_____

The thing I'm most proud of myself this week is: _____
_____
_____

I have noticed the seven pitfall thought patterns (personalization, pervasive-ness, paralysis-analysis, pessimism, polarization, psychic, permanence):

INCREASED   DECREASED   REMAINED THE SAME

I have felt the seven booster attributes (purpose, peace, pride, power, pas-sion, productivity, pleasure) in my life:

INCREASED   DECREASED   REMAINED THE SAME

Overall, I'm feeling: _____
_____
_____

Day 15, Week 3

Circle your maximum of 3 servings of pitfall foods.

Breakfast _____

_____

Lunch _____

_____

Dinner _____

_____

Snack (optional) _____

Snack (optional) _____

Snack (optional) _____

Booster activity 1 _____

_____

Booster activity 2 _____

_____

Booster activity 3 _____

_____

Day 16, Week 3

Circle your maximum of 3 servings of pitfall foods.

Breakfast _____

_____

Lunch _____

_____

Dinner _____

_____

Snack (optional) _____
Snack (optional) _____
Snack (optional) _____

Booster activity 1 _____

_____

Booster activity 2 _____

_____

Booster activity 3 _____

_____

Day 17, Week 3

Circle your maximum of 3 servings of pitfall foods.

Breakfast _____

_____

Lunch _____

_____

Dinner _____

_____

Snack (optional) _____

Snack (optional) _____

Snack (optional) _____

Booster activity 1 _____

_____

Booster activity 2 _____

_____

Booster activity 3 _____

_____

Day 18, Week 3

Circle your maximum of 3 servings of pitfall foods.

Breakfast _____

_____

Lunch _____

_____

Dinner _____

_____

Snack (optional) _____

Snack (optional) _____

Snack (optional) _____

Booster activity 1 _____

_____

Booster activity 2 _____

_____

Booster activity 3 _____

_____

Day 19, Week 3

Circle your maximum of 3 servings of pitfall foods.

Breakfast _____

_____

Lunch _____

_____

Dinner _____

_____

Snack (optional) _____

Snack (optional) _____

Snack (optional) _____

Booster activity 1 _____

_____

Booster activity 2 _____

_____

Booster activity 3 _____

_____

Day 20, Week 3

Circle your maximum of 3 servings of pitfall foods.

Breakfast _____
_____

Lunch _____
_____

Dinner _____
_____

Snack (optional) _____
Snack (optional) _____
Snack (optional) _____

Booster activity 1 _____
_____

Booster activity 2 _____
_____

Booster activity 3 _____
_____

Day 21, Week 3

Circle your maximum of 3 servings of pitfall foods.

Breakfast _____

_____

Lunch _____

_____

Dinner _____

_____

Snack (optional) _____

Snack (optional) _____

Snack (optional) _____

Booster activity 1 _____

_____

Booster activity 2 _____

_____

Booster activity 3 _____

_____

My weight: _____ **pounds**

What I learned about myself this week was: _____
_____
_____

What I think I need more of in my life is: _____
_____
_____

The thing I'm most proud of myself this week is: _____
_____
_____

I have noticed the seven pitfall thought patterns (personalization, pervasiveness, paralysis-analysis, pessimism, polarization, psychic, permanence):

INCREASED   DECREASED   REMAINED THE SAME

I have felt the seven booster attributes (purpose, peace, pride, power, passion, productivity, pleasure) in my life:

INCREASED   DECREASED   REMAINED THE SAME

Overall, I'm feeling: _____
_____
_____

287

Day 22, Week 4

Circle your maximum of 2 servings of pitfall foods.

Breakfast _____

_____

Lunch _____

_____

Dinner _____

_____

Snack (optional) _____

Snack (optional) _____

Snack (optional) _____

Booster activity 1 _____

_____

Booster activity 2 _____

_____

Booster activity 3 _____

_____

Booster activity 4 _____

_____

Day 23, Week 4

Circle your maximum of 2 servings of pitfall foods.

Breakfast _____

_____

Lunch _____

_____

Dinner _____

_____

Snack (optional) _____

Snack (optional) _____

Snack (optional) _____

Booster activity 1 _____

_____

Booster activity 2 _____

_____

Booster activity 3 _____

_____

Booster activity 4 _____

_____

Day 24, Week 4

Circle your maximum of 2 servings of pitfall foods.

Breakfast _____

_____

Lunch _____

_____

Dinner _____

_____

Snack (optional) _____

Snack (optional) _____

Snack (optional) _____

Booster activity 1 _____

_____

Booster activity 2 _____

_____

Booster activity 3 _____

_____

Booster activity 4 _____

_____

Day 25, Week 4

Circle your maximum of 2 servings of pitfall foods.

Breakfast _____

_____

Lunch _____

_____

Dinner _____

_____

Snack (optional) _____

Snack (optional) _____

Snack (optional) _____

Booster activity 1 _____

_____

Booster activity 2 _____

_____

Booster activity 3 _____

_____

Booster activity 4 _____

_____

Day 26, Week 4

Circle your maximum of 2 servings of pitfall foods.

Breakfast _____

_____

Lunch _____

_____

Dinner _____

_____

Snack (optional) _____

Snack (optional) _____

Snack (optional) _____

Booster activity 1 _____

_____

Booster activity 2 _____

_____

Booster activity 3 _____

_____

Booster activity 4 _____

_____

Day 27, Week 4

Circle your maximum of 2 servings of pitfall foods.

Breakfast _____

_____

Lunch _____

_____

Dinner _____

_____

Snack (optional) _____

Snack (optional) _____

Snack (optional) _____

Booster activity 1 _____

_____

Booster activity 2 _____

_____

Booster activity 3 _____

_____

Booster activity 4 _____

_____

Day 28, Week 4

Circle your maximum of 2 servings of pitfall foods.

Breakfast _____

_____

Lunch _____

_____

Dinner _____

_____

Snack (optional) _____

Snack (optional) _____

Snack (optional) _____

Booster activity 1 _____

_____

Booster activity 2 _____

_____

Booster activity 3 _____

_____

Booster activity 4 _____

_____

My weight: _____ **pounds**

What I learned about myself this week was: _____
_____
_____

What I think I need more of in my life is: _____
_____
_____

The thing I'm most proud of myself this week is: _____
_____
_____

I have noticed the seven pitfall thought patterns (personalization, pervasive-ness, paralysis-analysis, pessimism, polarization, psychic, permanence):

INCREASED   DECREASED   REMAINED THE SAME

I have felt the seven booster attributes (purpose, peace, pride, power, pas-sion, productivity, pleasure) in my life:

INCREASED   DECREASED   REMAINED THE SAME

Overall, I'm feeling: _____
_____
_____

Congratulations!

Be proud of yourself! You have made it through the 28-day Diet Rehab. You have probably figured out by now that my true wish for you is to keep living the principles you have learned here for the rest of your life. And now—through your own experience—you know what it *feels like* to fill your plate, your day, and your life with boosters. I hope you now realize that living this way is not a chore, because feeling good becomes the positive reinforcement that keeps you moving in an upward spiral that can easily last the rest of your life. Buy a notebook to use as your food journal or download one into your phone and continue to take care of yourself by engaging in booster activities every day.

My ultimate hope for you is to create so many affirming and boosting relationships, experiences, and activities that food is exactly what it should be: the delicious fuel that helps you live a rich, purpose-filled life.

7 Days of Quick
and Easy Recipes

Once you have reached week 3 of Diet Rehab, your brain has become balanced, which means you can begin to combine both serotonin and dopamine boosters to create delicious meals. These simple twenty-minute recipes—or sometimes restaurant orders—will help you to maintain a healthy balance of brain chemicals, keeping you both happy and healthy.

You can find more quick and easy recipes at
www.drmikedow.com.

---

7 Booster Breakfasts

The All-American: Mist a nonstick pan with olive oil spray. Whip 2 eggs or egg whites with a splash of skim milk, then add to the pan and scramble until light and fluffy, and season with a little black pepper. Mix in herbs such as thyme or basil at the last minute. Serve with 2 pieces of veggie or turkey sausage or bacon and 2 pieces of whole-wheat toast with a little olive oil or trans-fat-free spread. You could also have oatmeal instead of toast. Add some fresh cut melon and berries and coffee with a little skim milk.

Elated Egg Wrap: Mist a nonstick pan with olive oil spray. Whip 2 eggs or egg whites with a splash of skim milk, then add to the pan and scramble with low-fat cheese and some black pepper until light and fluffy. Top with fresh cut tomatoes, salsa, hot sauce, or herbs to taste. Wrap in a whole-wheat tortilla.

Berry High Protein: Mix 1 cup low-fat plain Greek yogurt with frozen (or fresh) blueberries, raspberries, or strawberries. Add a touch of xylitol to taste. Late to work? Put these ingredients in the blender with a little skim milk and throw it in a travel mug.

Eggs-on-the-Run: Mist a mug with olive oil spray. Fill the mug to the top with loose spinach, some sliced mushrooms, and diced tomatoes. Microwave on high for 15 seconds. Lightly beat 2 eggs or egg whites and add to the mug. Microwave on high for 50 seconds. Remove and stir. Microwave on high for another 50 seconds. Season with black pepper, dried herbes de Provence (fennel, basil, and thyme), or fresh herbs like chives, basil, or thyme.

Cinnaberry Oatmeal: Cook 1 packet of instant plain oatmeal in the microwave (or better yet, cook coarse-cut oats on the stove) with water, skim milk, unflavored soy milk, or unsweetened almond milk. Add in ½ banana, frozen (or fresh) blueberries, cinnamon, and—if you're craving a little sweet—xylitol. For an extra dopamine boost, stir in some vanilla whey protein. This goes great with black or green tea.

Butter My Muffin: Toast a whole-wheat muffin and spread it with 2 tablespoons of almond butter. If you're feeling like a sweet kick, add some banana slices. Coffee in a travel mug and you're out the door!

Brain-Booster Pancakes: Mix ¾ cup oatmeal, ½ cup low-fat cottage cheese, ⅛ teaspoon nutmeg, ⅛ teaspoon cinnamon, 1 teaspoon vanilla extract, 1 egg or 2 egg whites, and 1 cup skim milk in the blender. For an extra boost, add some blueberries and ½ banana. Cook as you would any pancake. Instead of butter and maple syrup, add some fresh berries, bananas, and cinnamon on top to sweeten. Or try a trans-fat-free spread like Flora Light.

7 Booster Lunches

Going Fishing: Take tuna in water or wild salmon (my favorites are John West or Princes wild-caught canned pink salmon). Stir in low-fat mayonnaise, a little mustard, and some chopped celery, apple, and walnuts. Take a piece of low-fat cheese, some crunchy romaine lettuce or sprouts, a sliced tomato, and put it all on toasted whole-wheat bread. Take the rest of the apple and cut it up for a side dish.

Peaceful Protein Pasta: Cook 2 ounces Barilla Plus pasta (high protein and high fiber) or whole-wheat pasta and drain. Mist a pan with olive oil spray and sauté your favorite green vegetables (think spinach, courgette, kale) with some garlic until just soft, then add marinara sauce. Add cooked turkey or 95% lean beef for a protein boost. Toss the sauce with your pasta, making sure that two-thirds of your dish is super-boosting veggies and protein and one-third pasta. Sprinkle with low-fat mozzarella, basil, and oregano. Serve with a piece of whole-wheat bread sprayed with a little bit of extra-virgin olive oil and drizzled with balsamic vinegar.

Keeping-You-Content Quinoa: Place ½ cup of quinoa in a pot with 1 cup water, frozen edamame, and some of your favorite frozen or fresh vegetables. Bring to a boil, then reduce the heat, cover, and simmer for 15 minutes. Season with balsamic vinegar and add 1 tablespoon of extra-virgin olive oil. Make a little extra for a great side dish for dinner!

Cheery Chicken Salad: In a large bowl, mix romaine lettuce, grilled chicken breast, chopped tomatoes, ½ avocado, shaved almonds, and apple slices. Add 1 tablespoon extra-virgin olive oil, a generous drizzle of balsamic vinegar, and black pepper to taste.

Joyous Jaunt: Okay, so you're on a road trip or have fifteen minutes to grab lunch. Bypass the burger joint for Subway. Order a 6-inch or 12-inch turkey, ham, grilled chicken, or veggie delight sandwich on omega-3 or whole-wheat bread with no cheese. Ask for the bread shelled out to maximize the super-boosting protein and veggies. Skip the iceberg lettuce and go for spinach. Ask for liberal amounts of tomato, green peppers, olives, onions, and jalapeños. Pour on the black pepper, mustard, and vinegar while skipping the mayonnaise, salt, and oil. Grab a bag of cut apples instead of crisps.

AB&B: Spread a couple tablespoons of almond butter on toasted whole-wheat bread. Skip the jam and slice ½ banana instead. Serve with a side of sliced carrots with hummus, celery, and salsa, or for a sweeter option, a whole apple or pear.

Seductive Soup and Salad: Pick any vegetable-based, non-creamy soup. My favorite restaurant options are Covent Garden Moroccan Tagine Soup or Hearty Vegetable. Pair with a crouton-free salad in a vinaigrette dressing—grilled chicken optional. If you're on the go, try Pret A Manger's chicken and avocado or tuna niçoise salad. Finish with a whole apple, orange, peach, or pear.

7 Booster Dinners

Pep-Me-Up Pizza: Take a whole-wheat pizza base or a whole-wheat tortilla, top with marinara sauce, low-fat mozzarella cheese, fresh oregano, fresh garlic, fresh basil, and your favorite cut vegetables, such as tomato slices, baby broccoli, olives, or artichoke. For an extra boost, add grilled chicken, shrimp, or veggie meat. Bake until everything is warm, bubbling, and smelling delicious.

Frickin' Happy Fried Rice: This is a great recipe to make if you have leftover brown rice in the fridge. Add ½ to 1 cup per person to a frying pan with just a couple tablespoons of olive oil. Add 2 eggs (or egg whites) per person and 1 to 2 cups of boosting vegetables to the mix: carrots, corn, peas, shredded broccoli, artichoke, and onion are all good options. Cook until all is warmed through and the eggs are cooked. Top it off with sesame seeds, a splash of low-sodium soy sauce, turmeric, and—for a dopamine boost—hot Thai sauce. (If you find yourself at your local Chinese dive, go for the grilled Szechuan chicken over the breaded orange variety. Skip the white rice and ask for extra grilled veggies with the sauce on the side, or do a half cup of brown rice.)

Titillating Tacos: Take a few grilled chicken breast strips, shrimp, or 95% lean beef and place on soft white sprouted corn or whole-wheat tortillas with low-fat cheese, lots of salsa, and fat-free sour cream. Skip the rice and go for a double serving of trans-fat-free pinto beans. For vegetarians, use the pinto beans for a taco filling. Garnish with fresh coriander, chopped fresh chile peppers, or hot sauce.

Marvelous Mac and Cheese: Cook 2 ounces Barilla Plus or whole-wheat pasta per person and strain. Toss with grilled baby broccoli, grilled chicken, and ¼ cup reduced-fat or fat-free cheese and 1 table-spoon of extra-virgin olive oil. Season with cracked black pepper and a few basil leaves.

Blissful Burger and Fries: Bake your favorite veggie burger patty, tur-key patty, or 95% lean beef patty and add slices of tomato and low-fat cheese, if desired. Put on a whole-wheat bun or wrap in romaine let-tuce. Go very light on the ketchup and heavy on the mustard or spicy mustard. Coat sweet potato strips in a little olive oil with a sprinkling of paprika and black pepper and bake for 20 minutes at 230°C/450°F. For dessert: nonfat Greek yogurt with frozen mixed berries and xylitol.

High-Spirit Steak, Sweet Potato, and Veg: Cook yourself your favorite filet mignon or other extra-lean beef. Flavor with your favorite herbs and spices. Pierce the skin of a small sweet potato or yam and bake for 45 minutes at 230°C/450°F. Sprinkle with cinnamon and trans-fat-free spread like Flora Light. Steam, grill, or sauté your favorite vegetables, such as broccoli, asparagus, or cauliflower in olive oil, garlic, and herbs. Have some orange slices or a whole pear for dessert.

Awesome Aubergine: Dip slices of aubergine in egg, then coat in whole-wheat bread crumbs (use 1 aubergine and 1 egg for every 2 serv-ings). Place on a baking sheet and bake at 230°C/450°F for about 5 minutes on each side. Then put your favorite marinara sauce in a baking dish and place the aubergine on top. Top with fresh oregano, basil, and low-fat mozzarella cheese, and bake for another 20 minutes. For dessert, have a decaf espresso and 2 squares of dark chocolate.

7 Booster Snacks

Not-So-Sinful Celery and Salsa: If there's one food that you *can* eat mindlessly while watching TV, this is it. (Of course, I always recommend mindful eating at a table whenever possible, but sometimes you just have to munch.)

Heavenly Hummus with Carrots and Tomatoes: I eat this snack so much that my dog Rocco now counts baby carrots as one of his favorite foods, too. Have baby carrots and cherry tomatoes in the fridge at all times. Keep them on a nice-looking platter and pretty soon even your kids will have no choice but to swap neon cheese puffs for these red and orange booster foods.

Fantastic Fruit Salad: Again, presentation is key. An apple sitting on the counter may look boring next to that multicolored bag of crisps, but when you slice and arrange a colorful platter of apples, grapes, blueberries, melon, and strawberries (with a sprinkle of lemon juice to keep the color), you're now using the Jedi mind trick that big food companies have been using on *you* all these years!

Fun and Frozen: My favorite and easiest snack is frozen grapes or frozen bananas. Throw washed grapes on a plate or in small plastic bags for a snack to take with you. When your bananas are turning a little black, that's the perfect time to peel, wrap in plastic wrap, and throw in the freezer.

Dopadelicious: Make a whey, casein, or soy-protein shake. Try different combinations blended with whole fruit, and use water, skim milk, or unsweetened almond milk. Pour them into ice cube trays with toothpicks. When you're in need of an afternoon snack that will keep you going, reach for one of these instead of that ice cream sandwich.

Crack-Me-Up: Have 4 or 5 of your favorite whole-wheat crackers such as Carr's Whole Wheat Crackers or Ryvita Whole Grain Rye Crispbread. Top with slices of low-fat cheese for a serotonin and dopamine booster snack.

My Mood Is Poppin': Air-pop popcorn and mist with a little extra-virgin olive oil. Or find a low-fat microwave variety (read the label and make sure there are no partially hydrogenated oils or trans fats). Pair with a whole apple, and you'll be satisfied till dinner.

APPENDIX B

Exceptions: Who Should *Not* Use Diet Rehab

There are several conditions that Diet Rehab is not intended to address, and many circumstances in which it should be used only under a physician's or psychotherapist's supervision. Please read the following section carefully if you have any of the following conditions:

- anorexia or bulimia
- excessive thinness: Body Mass Index below 18
- major depression or anxiety
- concerns about alcohol or drug use
- diabetes, on medication, or other health concerns

Anorexia or Bulimia

This book is not for you if you are experiencing anorexia or bulimia. If you're struggling with either one of these conditions, please seek help from your physician. These serious eating disorders are characterized by severe self-starvation and a cycle of bingeing and purging, either through self-inflicted vomiting or use of laxatives. Diet Rehab is not designed to treat these potentially life-threatening eating disorders. Conditions such as anorexia and bulimia can result in serious long-term health problems or even death, so please, if you suspect that you or a loved one is suffering from one of these illnesses, get professional help.

Excessive Thinness: Body Mass Index of 18 or Under

Similarly, if you are seeking to lose weight and are already too thin, with a BMI of 18 or under, you should not be following any weight-loss plan but should consult a professional to be screened for anorexia. You should use Diet Rehab only under the supervision of licensed health professionals and only in order to create new, healthier eating habits, not to lose weight.

For help locating an eating disorder treatment center, go to www .drmikedow.com.

Major Depression or Anxiety

If you are significantly depressed or anxious—feeling helpless, hopeless, suicidal, frequently tearful, noticing significant changes in sleep patterns or appetite, experience panic attacks, or insomnia—you need to consult your physician before starting this program. Although Diet Rehab may be helpful to you, you need first to rule out severe depression and anxiety, which may require medication and the supervision of a physician and/or psychotherapist. Diet Rehab is not designed to substitute for any medication your physician has prescribed for you.

Concerns About Drinking or Legal/Illegal Drugs

If you are struggling with an effort to contain your drinking or use of drugs you should first seek help with that issue. Consult your physician or consult my website—www.drmikedow.com—for treatment referrals for alcoholism and drug addiction.

Diabetes, on Medication, or Other Health Concerns

Finally, if you are a diabetic, on medication, or have any other health concerns, you must first seek the advice of your physician before beginning any weight-loss plan.

ACKNOWLEDGMENTS

First and foremost, thank you to my family, who always taught me that building a life filled with purpose and love is more important than material things. Mom, you never let me forget how loved I am, and even as a grown man, my freezer is still filled with healthy soups and casseroles you've made to prove it. Dad, I guess your lectures about me eating right paid off. David, your courage in the face of adversity makes you my hero and has given me some of the compassion I've needed to do my job every day. Grandpa, the cookies you've been baking and sending to me for years are still my favorite dessert—even though you'll understand why I've had to give some of them away after you read this book. Grandma, the love you showed me will always be with me.

To my television agent, Babette Perry, you took a leap of faith on me because you sensed I was a "good person." For that I will always be grateful. To my literary agent, Celeste Fine, you took a book that other agents would have thrown to the wolves and helped shape it like Michelangelo, skillfully carving away the excess marble to reveal the fine work underneath. Antonia Blyth, my brilliant cowriter, thank you for your talent and for countless hours of both on- and off-topic conversation that culminated in this book, and thanks to Heather Case and Reagan Alexander for bringing us together. To Rachel Kranz, thanks for helping carve. Thanks also to the amazing Lisa Lynch. To Andrew Strauser, Colin Whelan, Jennifer Williams, and everyone at TLC and Shed Media, thank you for a television show that helps me fulfill my life's calling. To my publicist Annie Jeeves, thanks for always promoting me in ways that are congruent with this calling. To everyone at Avery, thank you for your passion and vision. Thanks especially to my exceptional editor, Rachel Holtzman, who—case in point—got off a bus to plug in her phone at a rest stop to ensure that we'd work together (I'm very glad you did), and who, with genius and grace, guided the skillful execution of this book every step and revision along the way.

Thank you to everyone who has influenced my clinical work: Dr Mike Carragher, Dr Shannon Hanrahan, Dr Luis Rubalcava, Dr Diane Gehart, Dr Harville Hendrix, the entire staff at The Body Well integrative medical center, the Betty Ford Center, and Mark Smith. To all of my patients who shared the most intimate parts of their lives with me and allowed me to be a part of their healing journey: I hope your collective experience will help others who are on similar paths. To my friends who have been my second family in Los Angeles for over a decade, you have given me the confidence I needed to take big risks in my life; thanks for answering those calls in the wee hours of the morning.

God, you have given me so many blessings that I'm sometimes left in awe. Help me to always be an instrument of your peace and to make this world a better—and healthier—place.

BIBLIOGRAPHY

GENERAL READING

Amen, Daniel G. *Change Your Brain, Change Your Body*. Random House, 2010.

Bartz, Andrea. "Watered-Down Thinking." *Psychology Today* (February 2011): 36–37.

Beck, A. T., et al. *Cognitive Therapy of Depression*. Guilford Press, 1979.

Beckley, J., and H. R. Moskowitz. *Databasing the Consumer Mind: The Crave It!, Drink It!, Buy It! & Healthy You! Databases*. Institute of Food Technologists annual meeting, Anaheim, California, July 2002.

Brownell, K., and K. B. Horgen. *Food Fight: The Inside Story of the Food Industry, America's Obesity Crisis, and What We Can Do About It*. McGraw-Hill, 2003.

Challem, Jack. "Sunshine for Your Mind." *Nutrition Reporter*, 2002.

Cloninger, Robert C., et al. "Promotion of Well-Being in Person-Centered Mental Health Care." *Focus* 8 (Spring 2010): 165–79.

Ellis, Albert, with Russell Grieger et al. *Handbook of Rational-Emotive Therapy*. Springer Publishing, 1977.

Freedman, David H. "How to Fix the Obesity Crisis." *Scientific American* (February 2011).

Hart, Carol. *Secrets of Serotonin*. Book Associates, 1996.

Hyman, S. E. "Why Does the Brain Prefer Opium to Broccoli?" *Harvard Review of Psychiatry* (May–June 1994).

Kabat-Zinn, Jon. *Full Catastrophe Living: Using the Wisdom of Your Body and Mind to Face Stress, Pain, and Illness*. Random House, 1990.

Katherine, Anne. *Anatomy of a Food Addiction: An Effective Program to Overcome Compulsive Eating*. Gurze Books, 1996.

Kessler, David. *The End of Overeating*. Rodale, 2009.

Pecoraro, N., et al. "Chronic Stress Promotes Palatable Feeding, Which Reduces Signs of Stress: Feedforward and Feedback Effects of Chronic Stress." *Endocrinology* 145, no. 8 (August 1, 2004): 3754–62.

Pratt, Steven, and Kathy Matthews. *SuperFoods Rx: Fourteen Foods That Will Change Your Life*. HarperCollins, 2003.

Roizen, Michael F., and Mehmet C. Oz. *You, On a Diet: The Owner's Manual for Waist Management*. Free Press, 2006.

Seligman, Martin E. P. *Learned Optimism: How to Change Your Mind and Your Life*. Simon & Schuster, 1998.

Sheppard, Kay. *Food Addiction: The Body Knows*. Health Communications, 1993.

———. "The Science of Refined Food Addiction." *Counselor*, 2009.

Silver, Julie K. *Super Healing: The Clinically Proven Plan to Maximize Recovery from Illness or Injury*. Rodale, 2007.

Skinner, B. F. *About Behaviorism*. Vintage, 1974.

Somer, Elizabeth. *Eat Your Way to Happiness*. Harlequin, 2009.

Volkow, N. D., et al. "Overlapping Neuronal Circuits in Addiction and Obesity: Evidence of Systems Pathology." *Philosophical Transactions of the Royal Society: Biological Sciences* 363, no. 1507 (October 12, 2008): 3191–200.

Wise, R. A. "The Role of Reward Pathways in the Development of Drug Dependence." *Pharmacology and Therapeutics* 35, no. 1–2 (1987): 227–63.

Wurtman, J. "Dropping Serotonin Levels: Why You Crave Carbs Late in the Day." *Huffington Post*, February 16, 2011.

INTRODUCTION: HOW I KICKED MY FOOD ADDICTION . . . AND HOW YOU CAN, TOO

Guertin, T. L., and A. J. Conger. "Mood and Forbidden Foods' Influence on Perceptions of Binge Eating." *Addictive Behaviors* 24, no. 2 (March 4, 1999): 175–93.

Kenny, Paul J., and Paul M. Johnson. "Addiction-Like Reward Dysfunction and Compulsive Eating in Obese Rats: Role for Dopamine D2 Receptors." *Nature Neuroscience* 13 (2010): 635–41.

Leibowitz, S. F., and B. G. Hoebel. "Behavioral Neuroscience and Obesity." In *The Handbook of Obesity*. Edited by G. Bray, C. Bouchard, and P. James. Marcel Dekker, 2004.

Volkow, Nora D., and Roy A. Wise. *How Can Drug Addiction Help Us Understand Obesity*. Nature Publishing Group, 2005.

CHAPTER 1. WILLPOWER IS NOT THE PROBLEM

Agatston, Arthur. *The South Beach Diet*. Rodale, 2003.

Atkins, Robert C. *Dr Atkins' New Diet Revolution*. Simon & Schuster, 2002.

Avena, Nicole M., et al. "Evidence for Sugar Addiction: Behavioral and Neurochemical Effects of Intermittent, Excessive Sugar Intake." *Neuroscience and Biobehavioral Review* 32, no. 1 (2008): 20–39.

D'Adamo, Peter J., and Catherine Whitney. *Eat Right 4 Your Type: The Individualized*

Diet Solution to Staying Healthy, Living Longer & Achieving Your Ideal Weight. Putnam, 1996.

DeMaria, E. J., et al. "High Failure Rate After Laparoscopic Adjustable Silicone Gastric Banding for Treatment of Morbid Obesity." *Annals of Surgery* 233, no. 6 (June 2001): 809–18.

Elkins, Gary, et al. "Noncompliance with Behavioral Recommendations Following Bariatric Surgery." *Obesity Surgery* 15, no. 4 (2005): 546–51.

Harmon, Katherine. "Addicted to Fat: Overeating May Alter the Brain as Much as Hard Drugs." *Scientific American* (March 28, 2010).

Kaufman, Frederick. "The Domino's Effect." *Men's Health,* November 9, 2010.

Kenny, Paul J., and Paul M. Johnson. "Addiction-Like Reward Dysfunction and Compulsive Eating in Obese Rats: Role for Dopamine D2 Receptors." *Nature Neuroscience* 13 (2010:) 635–41.

Wang, G. J., et al. "Exposure to Appetitive Food Stimuli Markedly Activates the Human Brain." *NeuroImage* 21, no. 4 (April 2004): 1790–97.

———. "Similarity Between Obesity and Drug Addiction as Assessed by Neurofunctional Imaging: A Concept Review." *Journal of Addictive Diseases* 23, no. 3 (2004): 39–53.

CHAPTER 2. HOW FOOD ADDICTION MAKES YOU FAT

Allison, D. B., M. S. Faith, and J. S. Nathan. "Risch's Lambda Values for Human Obesity." *International Journal of Obesity and Related Metabolic Disorders* 20, no. 11 (1996): 990–99.

Arias-Carrión, O., and E. Pöppel. "Dopamine, Learning and Reward-Seeking Behavior." *Acta Neurobiologiae Experimentalis* (Warsaw) 67, no. 4 (2007): 481–88.

Bouchard, C., et al. "Inheritance of the Amount and Distribution of Human Body Fat." *International Journal of Obesity* 12, no. 3 (1988): 205–15.

Epel, E. S., et al. "Stress and Body Shape: Stress-Induced Cortisol Secretion Is Consistently Greater Among Women with Central Fat." *Psychosomatic Medicine* (September/October 2000).

Farooqi, I. S., et al. "Clinical Spectrum of Obesity and Mutations in the Melanocortin 4 Receptor Gene." *New England Journal of Medicine* 348, no. 12 (March 2003).

Lee, J. H., D. R. Reed, and R. A. Price. "Familial Risk Ratios for Extreme Obesity: Implications for Mapping Human Obesity Genes." *International Journal of Obesity* 21, no. 10 (October 1997): 935–40.

Le Magnen, J. "A Role for Opiates in Food Reward and Food Addiction." In *Taste, Experience, and Feeding.* Edited by P. T. Capaldi. American Psychological Association, 1990.

Shengxu, Li, et al. "Physical Activity Attenuates the Genetic Predisposition to Obesity in 20,000 Men and Women from EPIC-Norfolk Prospective Population Study." *PLoS Medicine* (August 2010).

Stice, Eric, et al. "Obesity, Abnormal Reward Circuitry in Brain Linked: Gene Tied to Dopamine Signaling Also Implicated in Overeating." *ScienceDaily* (October 17, 2008).

Stunkard, A. J., et al. "The Body-Mass Index of Twins Who Have Been Reared Apart." *New England Journal of Medicine* 322, no. 21 (May 24, 1990): 1483–87.

Swift, Robert M. "Medications and Alcohol Craving." *Alcohol Research and Health* 23 (1999).

Tambs, K., et al. "Genetics and Environmental Contributions to the Variance of the Body Mass Index in a Norwegian Sample of First-Degree and Second-Degree Relatives." *American Journal of Human Biology* 3 (1991): 257–68.

Vogler, G. P., et al. "Influences of Genes and Shared Family Environment on Adult Body Mass Index Assessed in an Adoption Study by a Comprehensive Path Model." *International Journal of Obesity and Related Metabolic Disorders* 19, no. 1 (January 1995): 40–45.

Wang, G. J., et al. "Brain Dopamine and Obesity." *The Lancet* 357 (2001): 354–57.

Wansink, B., et al. "Internal and External Cues: French and American Explanations for Mindless Eating." *FASEB Journal* 20 (2006): A175–76.

CHAPTER 3. THE SECRET OF GRADUAL DETOX

Ellis, Albert, Russell Grieger, et al. *Handbook of Rational-Emotive Therapy.* Springer Publishing, 1977.

Simmons, Garey. "Are You a Little Low on Serotonin or Dopamine?" *Ezinearticles* (December 2007).

Spudich, Tiffany. "Cortisol and Weight." *Project Aware* (January 2007).

CHAPTER 4. FEELING ANXIOUS: HUNGRY FOR SEROTONIN

Anderson, I. M., et al. "Dieting Reduces Plasma Tryptophan and Alters Brain 5-HT Function in Women." *Psychological Medicine* 20, no. 4 (November 1990): 785–91.

Benwell, M. E., D. J. Balfour, and J. M. Anderson. "Smoking-Associated Changes in the Serotonergic Systems of Discrete Regions of Human Brain." *Psychopharmacology* (Berlin) 102, no. 1 (1990): 68–72.

Blass, E., E. Fitzgerald, and P. Kehoe. "Interactions Between Sucrose, Pain and Isolation Distress." *Pharmacology, Biochemistry and Behavior* 26, no. 3 (March 1987): 483–89.

Denmark, F. L., and M. A. Paludi. *Psychology of Women.* Greenwood Press, 1993.

Formanek, R., and A. Gurian. *Women and Depression: A Lifespan Perspective.* Springer, 1987.

"Get Angry When Hungry? Blame Low Serotonin." Reuters, June 30, 2008.

Holt, S. H., J. C. Miller, and P. Petocz. "Interrelationships Among Postprandial Satiety, Glucose and Insulin Responses and Changes in Subsequent Food Intake." *European Journal of Clinical Nutrition* (December 1996).

Lyubomirsky, Sonja. *The How of Happiness—A New Approach to Getting the Life You Want.* Penguin Press, 2007.

Peciña, S., et al. "Hyperdopaminergic Mutant Mice Have Higher 'Wanting' but Not 'Liking' for Sweet Rewards." *Journal of Neuroscience* 23, no. 28 (October 15, 2003): 9395–402.

Pick, Marcelle. "An Introduction to Insulin Resistance." Womentowomen.com, 2004.

Saito, H., et al. "Psychological Factors That Promote Behavior Modification by Obese Patients." *BioPsychoSocial Medicine* (September 2009).

Stokes, Christina, and Jeremy Watson. "Why Lighting Up Always Gets You Down." *Scotland on Sunday,* March 14, 2004.

Weissman, M. M., and E. S. Paykel. *The Depressed Woman.* University of Chicago Press, 1974.

Wiley, T. S., and Bent Formby. *Lights Out: Sleep, Sugar, and Survival.* Simon & Schuster, 2001.

Wurtman, Judith J., and Nina Frusztajer Marquis. *The Serotonin Power Diet.* Rodale, 2006.

Yu, Winnie. "A Losing Personality." *Scientific American Mind* (January/February 2011).

CHAPTER 5. FEELING BLUE: RAVENOUS FOR DOPAMINE

Beckley, J., and H. R. Moskowitz. *Databasing the Consumer Mind: The Crave It!, Drink It!, Buy It! & Healthy You! Databases.* Institute of Food Technologists annual meeting, Anaheim, California, July 2002.

Brain, Marshall, and Charles W. Bryant. "How Caffeine Works." *Discovery Health* (April 2000).

Gramling, C. "Gender Gap: Male-Only Gene Affects Men's Dopamine Levels." *Science News* 169, no. 9 (March 1, 2006): 132–33.

Hemat., R. A. S. *Andropathy.* Urotext, 2007.

Kenny, Paul J., and Paul M. Johnson. "Addiction-Like Reward Dysfunction and Compulsive Eating in Obese Rats: Role for Dopamine D2 Receptors." *Nature Neuroscience* 13 (2010): 635–41.

Munro, C., et al. "Sex Differences in Striatal Dopamine Release in Healthy Adults." *Journal of Biological Psychiatry* 59, no. 10 (2006): 966–74.

Redgrave, Peter, and Kevin Gurney. "The Short-Latency Dopamine Signal: A Role in Discovering Novel Actions?" *Nature Reviews Neuroscience* 7 (December 2006): 967–75.

Stice, E., et al. "Relation Between Obesity and Blunted Striatal Response to Food Is Moderated by TaqIA A1 Allele." *Science* 322, no. 5900 (October 17, 2008): 449–52.

Volnow, N. D. "Evaluating Dopamine Reward Pathway in ADHD: Clinical Implications." *Journal of the American Medical Association* 302, no. 10 (September 9, 2009): 1084–91.

CHAPTER 6. FEELING POWERLESS: STARVING FOR EVERYTHING

Kabat-Zinn, Jon. *Wherever You Go, There You Are: Mindfulness Meditation in Everyday Life.* Hyperion, 1994.

CHAPTER 7. OBSESSIVE EATING: SEEKING SECURITY

Beyette, Beverly, and Jeffrey H. Schwartz. *Brain Lock: Free Yourself from Obsessive-Compulsive Behavior: A Four-Step Self-Treatment Method to Change Your Brain Chemistry.* ReganBooks, 1997.

Huppert, Jonathan, and Deborah Roth. "Treating Obsessive-Compulsive Disorder with Exposure and Response Prevention." *Behavior Analyst Today* (Winter 2003).

Neziroglu, Fugen, and Mani Anup. "Relationship of Eating Disorders to OCD." *OCD Chicago,* January 2009.

Sullivan, S., et al. "Personality Characteristics in Obesity and Relationship with Successful Weight Loss." *International Journal of Obesity* (April 1, 2007): 669–74.

CHAPTER 8. EMOTIONAL EATING: THE SEARCH FOR JOY

Albers, Susan. *50 Ways to Soothe Yourself Without Food.* New Harbinger, 2009.

Roth, Geneen. *Breaking Free from Emotional Eating.* Plume, 1993.

CHAPTER 9. BINGE EATING: REGAINING CONTROL

Fairburn, Christopher G. *Overcoming Binge Eating.* Guilford Press, 1995.

Quinlan, Kimberley. "Binge Eating Disorder / Compulsive Overeating and Its Treatment." *OCD Center of Los Angeles Blog,* November 16, 2010.

CHAPTER 10. CHANGE YOUR TASTES, CHANGE YOUR BODY

Bertino, M., G. K. Beauchamp, and K. Engelman. "Long-Term Reduction in Dietary Sodium Alters the Taste of Salt." *American Journal of Clinical Nutrition* 36 (1982): 1134–44.

Dinehart, M. E., et al. "Bitter Taste Markers Explain Variability in Vegetable Sweetness, Bitterness, and Intake." *Physiology & Behavior* 87 (2006): 304–13.

Drewnowski, A., S. A. Henderson, and A. Barratt-Fornell. "Genetic Taste Markers and Food Preferences." *Drug Metabolism and Disposition* 29, no. 4, part 2 (April 2001): 535–38.

Hayes, J. E. "Response to Lack of Relation Between Bitter Taste Receptor TAS2R38 and BMI in Adults." *Obesity* (October 2010).

Holt, S. H., et al. "A Satiety Index of Common Foods." *European Journal of Clinical Nutrition* 49, no. 9 (September 1995): 675–90.

Neergaard, Lauren. "Doctors Say How We Taste Affects Health." Associated Press, November 21, 2011.

CHAPTER 11. SALT JUNKIES: HOOKED ON THE GATEWAY DRUG

Hayes, J. E., B. S. Sullivan, and V. B. Duffy. "Explaining Variability in Sodium Intake Through Oral Sensory Phenotype, Salt Sensation and Liking." *Physiology and Behavior* 100, no. 4 (June 16, 2010): 369–80.

Hellmich, Nanci. "Consumers' Tastes Make It Difficult to Dash Salt from Diets." *USA Today,* April 28, 2010.

Institute of Medicine of the National Academies. "Strategies to Reduce Sodium Intake in the United States." Food and Nutrition Board consensus report, April 20, 2010.

Kessler, David A. *The End of Overeating.* Rodale, 2009.

CHAPTER 12. STARVED FOR SEROTONIN: JONESING FOR SUGAR AND CARBS

Albers, Susan. *50 Ways to Soothe Yourself Without Food.* New Harbinger, 2009.

CHAPTER 13. DOPAMINE-DEPRIVED: LONGING FOR FAT AND CAFFEINE

"Dopamine: Natural Ways to Increase Dopamine Levels." IntegrativePsychiatry.net.

Juhasz, Francine. "Foods That Affect Dopamine Levels in the Brain." Livestrong.com (February 2011).

Kelly, G. S. "Nutritional and Botanical Interventions to Assist with the Adaptation to Stress." *Alternative Medicine Review* (September 1999).

Melo, F. H., et al. "Antidepressant-like Effect of Carvacrol (5-Isopropyl-2-methylphenol) in Mice: Involvement of Dopaminergic System." *Fundamental & Clinical Pharmacology* 25, no. 3 (June 2011): 362–67.

Schrock, Karen. "Parsley, Sage, Rosemary and Thyme." *Scientific American Mind* (January/February 2011).

INDEX

Page numbers in italics refer to illustrations.

AB&B recipe, 300
ADD/ADHD, 111–13, 115–16
Adderall, 113
Addiction. *See* Food addiction
Adrenaline (epinephrine), 116
Agreeable personalities, 84
Alcohol, 237–38
The All-American, 297–98
Animal protein, 206, 220
Anorexia, 141, 144, 304
Antidepressants, 2, 11, 79, 83, 111
Anxiety, 59, 147, 305
   diet creating, 29
   fearful feelings, fearful actions and,
      88–89, *89*
   food addiction and, 3–5
   mantra and, *88, 95*
   perfectionism and, 5, 85–86, 93,
      201–2
   pitfall thought patterns and, 85–86,
      201–2
   serotonin and, 2, 78, 84–85, *85*, 101,
      142, 201
Atkins Diet, 22, 28, 181

Attitudes, and dopamine, serotonin
      levels, *128*, 128–29, 142
Awesome Aubergine, 302

Bariatric surgery, 25–26, 41–42
Beans, 206
Beliefs, *91*, 91–92, 121–22, *122*
Berry High Protein, 298
Betty Ford Center, 34
Binge eating, 7, 92, 167, 175, 178
   carbohydrates, sugar and fat for, 166
   cognitive-behavioral therapy for,
      167
   eating normal for weight loss, 170
   emotional reactions from, 170
   fear and, 168–69, 175
   graded exposure therapy for, 175
   hunger, 167, 172–73
   journal for, 175
   mantra changed in, 168
   quiz for, 171–72
   rules to live by, 176–78
   in secret, 168
   self-medication for, 170

Binge eating (*cont.*)
  serotonin, dopamine and, 166–67,
      170, 173, 174
  shame of, 167
  triggers of, 169, 173
  weight not related to, 174
Blame, 55–56
Blissful Burger and Fries, 301
Blood sugar, 80, 100
Blueberries, 233
The Body Well, 34
Booster activities, 6, 9, 47, 49, 155. *See
      also* Dopamine booster
      activities; Serotonin booster
      activities
  booster attributes targeted with, 63,
      133–34
  brain chemistry improved by, 92
Booster foods, 7, 156–57. *See also*
      Dopamine booster foods; Dual
      deficiency; Serotonin booster
      foods
  for anxiety, 85, 142
  binge eating improved by, 7, 92
  "buzz-crash" cycle eliminated by, 126
  cravings, healthy habits fostered by,
      93
  food addiction tackled by, 49, 129
  hunger and, 40
  for kitchen rehabbing, 190
  meals/snacks for, 231–32, 243,
      297–303
  satiety high from, 189, *189*
  self-medication with, 86, 115–16
  weight loss gradual, sustainable with,
      25, 93
Boosters, 8. *See also* Dopamine
      boosters; Mantra boosters;
      Serotonin boosters
  ADD/ADHD and, 115–16
  attributes, 63–67, *64*, 99, 133–34,
      161–63
  binge eating as, 167, 173, 174

brain chemistry improved by, 7,
      63–67, 92, 94
  Diet Rehab program for, 46–48, 49,
      85, 92, 100, 124, 202–4
  emotional eating patterns as,
      157–58, 160, 165
  endorphins as, 82
  for exhaustion, 115
  feelings helped by, 129
  gradual detox added as, 76
  replacing pitfalls, 46–48, 53, 81, 94,
      97–98, 117, 182–83, 240
  thought patterns for, 48, 53, 94,
      117
  thoughts, feelings changed, 92–93,
      96–97, 150
Brain-Booster Pancakes, 299
Brain chemistry, 2, 9–10
  balancing of, 18–20, 26
  bariatric surgery not improved with,
      25–26, 41–42
  binge eating and, 167
  boosters to improve, 7, 63–67, 92,
      94
  compulsive eating and, 22
  cravings and, 2, 6–7, 19–20
  Diet Rehab program and, 18–20, 24,
      26, 105, 170
  diets damaging to, 32, 37
  dopamine and, 2, 9, 18–20, 101,
      159
  emotional eating from, 2, 159–60
  exercise to improve, 38
  feel-good biochemicals, 2, 20, 82
  food addiction created by, 7, 15–16,
      30, 52
  gradual detox for healthy, 34
  high-fat and high-sugar diets
      damaging, 8, 15–16, 18–19
  mantra, influenced by, 119–20,
      131–34
  medication and, 33–34
  obesity and, 38

out-of-control feeling from imbalance, 129
pitfall activities reducing, 47
power of, 126
serotonin, dopamine and, 2, 9, 20, 71, 82, 159–60
Bulimia, 141–42, 144, 304
Butter My Muffin, 298
"Buzz-crash" cycle, 126

Caffeine, 113–14, 216
self-medication with, 115–16
Calories, 8, 152, 188–89, 239
Carbohydrates
binge eating of, 166
serotonin and, 2, 7, 21, 83, 150, 152, 201–2
tolerance of sugar and, 79
Cardiovascular system, 78–79
Challenge foods, 182–83
Cheery Chicken Salad, 299–300
Cigarettes/smoking, 82–83, 123–24, 126
Cinnaberry Oatmeal, 298
Cocaine, 189
Cognitive-behavioral therapy, 6, 9, 53, 167
Comfort food, 2, 21–22, 202
Compulsive eating, 13–14, 22
Concerta, 113
Control issues, 129, 142, 145–46, 151, 153, 157, 167
Cooking, 177, 237, 300
Cortisol, 36–37, 40, 113
Crack-Me-Up, 303
Cravings
brain chemistry and, 2, 6–7
for carbohydrates, sugar and starch, 100, 150, 201–2
cycle of, 19–20
dopamine and, 42–43, 105, 111–12, 216
for fat and caffeine, 126

habits, healthy replacing, 46, 93
recalibration of taste and, 183–85

Dairy, 205, 220
Depression, 305
dopamine shortage from, 2, 216
self-medicating, soda for, 115
vitamin D to help combat, 203
women and low serotonin, risk of, 83–84, 111
Desserts, 208, 223
Detachment, from emotional eating patterns, 161–62
Detox, gradual, 8, 10, 15, 34, 44, 192
addiction and, 24–25, 26, 46
boosters added to, 76
Diet Rehab program and, 24–26, 44–46, 50–52, 192, 231
unhealthy habits and, 45
withdrawal symptoms by, 45–46
Diabetes, 81, 238
Dieting, constant, 142
Diet Rehab Community, 236
Diet Rehab program, 17, 46–48, 49, 85, 92, 100, 124
anorexia and, 304
booster activities for, 231–32
booster foods for, 129, 231–32, 297–303
brain chemistry and, 24, 26, 105, 170
bulimia and, 304
calories in, 239
cognitive-behavioral therapy for, 53
contract of, 249–51
depression and, 305
dopamine, serotonin and, 232
dual deficiencies, regaining control with, 135–37
exercise in, 237
foods, 191–92
gradual detox plan for, 24–26, 45–46, 50–52, 192, 231

Diet Rehab program (*cont.*)
  habits, creating new, 25, 98
  health conditions not suitable for, 304–5
  journals for, 235, 252–63
  maintenance of, 234–35
  mantra transformed with, 90–92
  meals, 191–92
  pitfalls, 231, 240
  questions about, 236–42
  schedules, 233–34
  serotonin and, 100, 201, 202–4, 232
  treatment plan, 202–4
Diets, restrictive
  anxiety-creating, 29
  Atkins Diet, 22, 28, 181
  brain chemistry damage from, 32, 37
  counting calories, 8
  failure of, 22–23, 28–29, 32, 44–45, 181–82
  low carbohydrate, serotonin deprivation from, 83
  outside-in approach of, 48
  serotonin, dopamine depletion from, 24–25
  South Beach Diet, 22, 28, 181
  starvation mode from, 22–23
  weight gain with, 22–23, *23*, 24–25, *25*
  willpower and, 22
  women, problems with, 83–84
  the Zone, 28
Digestion, 79
Distraction, 57–58, 163, 177
Domino's, 26
Dopadelicious, 303
Dopamine
  bariatric surgery reducing levels of, 41–42
  behaviors, substances releasing, 102
  brain chemistry and, 2, 9, 18–20, 101, 159

caffeine and, 113, 216
cigarettes/smoking, boost and crash of, 82–83
cocaine high of, 189
cortisol, and depletion of, 36–37
depression and depletion of, 2
Dopamine-Deficient Food Journal, 256–259
drugs, boosting levels of, 2–3
energizing and crashing from, 2, 17–18
high-fat diet and, 2, 7, 103, *104*, 216
meals for, 223
men, low levels of, 110–11
natural production restored for, 124, 126
oxytocin interaction with, 101
restrictive diet and depletion of, 24–25
reward response of, 42–43, 111–12
sleep deprivation and, 113
withdrawal symptoms of, 17–18
women, low levels and weight gain, 112
Dopamine, high levels, 102, 126
Dopamine, low levels, 101–5
  ADD/ADHD from, 111, 112–13
  behaviors and, 104, *104*, *128*
  binge eating from, 166, 167, 170, 174
  cravings from, 105, 216
  depression from, 2, 216
  discouraged thoughts cycle of, 117, *117*
  emotional eating indicated by, 154, 159–60
  feelings created by, 101–3, 120, 217
  food addiction, weight gain from, 120
  high-fat diet and, 19, *19*, 22, 103–4, *104*
  mantra and, 117, *117*, 118–19, 122, *122*, 125, 127

pitfall thought patterns, increase of, 9, 54, *54*

ravenous with, 105–10, 118–19

self-medication with pitfall foods, 115–16, 216

sleep deprivation and, 113

Dopamine boosters, 6, 112, 124

Dopamine booster activities, 6, 125, 203, 217–19

list of, 223–28

mantra, for transforming, 85

upward spiral of, 122, *122*

Dopamine booster foods, 3, 24, 43, 112, 115–16, 117, 124–25

beans, 221

dairy, low-fat, 220

desserts, 223

drinks, 223

fruit, 222, 237

meals/snacks of, 243, 297–303

nuts, seeds, 221

oils and dressings, 222

proteins, 218, 220

seafood, 221

spices, herbs, 223

sweeteners, 223

vegetables, 222

whole grains, seeds, 220

Dopamine pitfall foods, 229

Drinking/drinks, 208, 223, 237–38, 305

Drugs, 2–3, 15, 305

Dual deficiency, 127–37

attitudes, behaviors of, *128*, 128–29

from binge eating, 166

booster foods added for, 129

Diet Rehab program and, 135–37

emotional eating from, 154

high-stress life from, 135

journals, 260–63

mantra and, 127, 130–31, 154

out-of-control feelings in, 129, *129*

starving for everything with, 127–37

weight gain by, 134

withdrawal more difficult with, 129–30

Dunkin' Donuts, 100

Ecstasy (MDMA), 2–3

Eggs-on-the-Run, 298

Elated Egg Wrap, 298

Emotional eating patterns

booster foods for, 157–58, 160, 165

brain chemistry cause of, 159–60

change created by changing experience, 160–61

from dual deficiency, 154

emotional challenges and, 157, 160

exercises for, 161–65

feeling full, learning to, 160

freedom, weight and, 154–57

overwhelming feelings of, 159

physical cause of, 160

pitfalls of, 154–56

quiz for, 158–59

serotonin, dopamine and, 159

triggers of, 155

Emotional reactions, 170

The End of Overeating (Kessler), 193

Endorphins, 82

Epinephrine. *See* Adrenaline

Exercise, 175

brain chemistry improved by, 38

Diet Rehab program and, 237

for hypertension, 198

for obesity, 38

obsessive, 142, 147, 152, 155

Exhaustion, 115

Fantastic Fruit Salad, 302

Fear, 142, 168–69, 175

Flavors, natural, 184

Food, 2. *See also* Booster foods; Meals; Pitfall foods; Recipes

accepting new, 98, 188

addictive, 1, 6, 7, 46, 189, 193

allergies for, 238

Food (*cont.*)
  avoidance of, 30
  brain chemistry interacting with, 2
  comfort, 2, 21–22
  deceptive marketing of, 100
  enjoyment of, 176
  family, healthy meals for, 191–92
  fear of, 142, 168–69, 175
  going public with, 168–69, 177–78
  obsessive relationship to, 142
  portion sizes, 204–5, 219–20
  salt, as gateway drug, 194
  self-medication with, 2, 5, 9, 29, 86,
      90, 115–16
  serotonin-releasing, 147
  tastes stimulated by salt, 193, 195
Food addiction, 1, 3, 193, 242
  ADD/ADHD vulnerable to, 113
  anxiety and, 3–5
  behavior of, 2, 29, 155
  booster foods and activities to help,
      49
  brain chemistry creating, 7, 15–16,
      30, 52
  causes of, 1–6, 146
  concealing, 6, 141
  dopamine and, 42–43, 103, 120
  drug addiction and, 15
  dual deficiency and, 135
  familiarity, stability sought from,
      147–48
  freedom from, 26, 27, 32
  gradual detox from, 24–25, 26, 46
  habits changing, 27, 142
  high-fat, high-sugar foods and,
      15–16, 26, 135
  hunger and, 40
  "layering" of salt, fat in snack foods,
      193
  medication for, 33–34
  neurochemical dependency of,
      15–17
  physical need of, 14, 30

pitfall foods, 48
quiz for, 30–32
rituals, obsessive eating, 145, 147,
    149, 152
satiety, low, 188–89
serotonin and, 89, 147
shame of, 13–14
stress and anxiety creating, 3–4
sugar and, 14, 35
tolerance creating, 32–33
weight and, 26, 28–30, 120
willpower and, 7, 14, 16, 30
withdrawal symptoms from, 14, 20,
    34–35, 79
yo-yo dieting and, 29
Freaky Eaters, 7, 9, 13
Frickin' Happy Fried Rice, 300–301
Friend, finding, 177
Frito-Lay, 193
Fruit, 207–8, 222, 237
Fun and Frozen, 302–3

Genetics, 38, 94–95
Ghrelin, 203
Gluten-free, 238
Goals, 174
Going Fishing, 299
Graded exposure therapy, 175
Gratitude, 57, 162, 164
Gum, 177, 240

Habits
  addictive food, changing, 27, 142
  cravings replaced by healthy, 46,
      93
  Diet Rehab program and, 25, 98
  new food, four weeks for, 98
  salt, breaking of, 195, 197–98
  soda, 114–15
Happiness gene, 94–95
*Heavenly Hummus with Carrots and
    Tomatoes*, 302
Herbs. *See* Spices, herbs

High-fat, high-sugar foods, 15–16, 26
High-fat diet, 35
    brain chemistry and, 8, 15–16,
        18–19
    dopamine and, 2, 7, 103–4, *104*,
        105, 216
    satiety, low, 188–89
    saturated fat in, 26, 228
    tolerance, cycle of, 19, *19*, 22
    weight gain from, 17
High-Spirit Steak, Sweet Potato, and Veg,
    301–2
Hunger
    binge eating and, 167, 172–73
    booster foods and, 40
    cortisol and, 40
    ghrelin, hunger hormone, 203
    quiz for, 39
    understanding, 40–41
Hypertension, 196, 198

Inside-out approach, 49
Insulin resistance
    blood sugar and, 80
    diabetes with, 81
    weight gain from, 36–37
Interventions, for food obsessions,
    145–53

Journals, 168–69, 176
    binge eating record for, 175
    Diet Rehab program, key to, 235,
        252–63
Joyous Jaunt, 300
Juice, 239

Keeping-You-Content Quinoa, 299
Kessler, David, 193
Kitchen rehab, 190
Kosher, 238

"Layering," of fat, salt in snack foods,
    193–94

Lean protein, 218
Love letters, 162

Mantra, 84–91
    actions, consequences and beliefs
        changed by, 91, 91–92, 121–22,
        122
    anxiety and, 88, 95
    "because" challenge, dopamine-
        boosting list of, 123–25
    "because" challenge, dual deficit list
        of, 131
    "because" challenge, serotonin-
        boosting list of, 93–94, 97
    binge eating and, 168
    booster attributes improving, 99
    brain chemistry and, 119–20, 131–34
    Diet Rehab program transforming,
        90–92
    dopamine and, 117, *117*, 118–19,
        122, *122*, 125, 127
    dual deficiency and, 127–37,
        130–31, 154
    emotional eating and, 154–56
    list of improved, 89–90, 120–21,
        130–31
    serotonin deficiency and, 87–88, 150
    weight influenced by, 87–88,
        119–20, 149
Mantra boosters, 85
    actions, thoughts and feelings
        changed with, 92–93, 96–97,
        150
    changing mantra pitfall to, 95–96,
        120–23, 130–31, 168
    dual deficiency choices of, 130–31
    for serotonin, 72, 92, *92*, 96, 100,
        208–13
Mantra pitfalls, 85–87, 95
    actions, consequences to transform,
        91, *91*, 96
    booster transforming from, 89–90,
        118–19

Mantra pitfalls (*cont.*)
 Diet Rehab program transforming,
  90–92
 dual deficiency of, 154
 identifying, 89, 90–91
 mantra boosters changing from,
  95–96, 120–23, 130–31, 168
 positive message replacing, 86–87,
  155–56, 168
 serotonin levels depleted by, 87–88,
  150
 weight and, 89, 149–50
Marvelous Mac and Cheese, 301
McDonald's, 100
Meals, 231–32
 binge eaters, rules to live by,
  176–78
 for Diet Rehab program, 191–92
 dopamine- and serotonin-boosting,
  243
 planning, 223
 recipes for booster, 297–303
Medication, 33–34
Meditation, 162, 168
Men
 ADD/ADHD and, 111, 112–13
 dopamine deprivation and, 110–11
 serotonin, higher levels in, 111
Metabolism, 38, 149
Migraines, 20
Mindful walking, 163
My Mood Is Poppin', 303

Neurochemical dependency, 15–17
Norepinephrine, 116
Not-So-Sinful Celery and Salsa, 302
Novelty-seeking personalities, 118
Nuts, seeds, 221

Obesity, 38, 118
Obsessive behaviors, 142, 143, 151,
  157
Obsessive-compulsive disorder, 78, 144

Obsessive eating, 141–53
 familiarity, stability sought from,
  147–48
 food rituals, 145, 147–48, 149, 152
 interventions for, 145–53
 quiz for, 143–44
 security, sought from, 141
 serotonin boosters for, 142, 145
Obsessive exercise, 142, 147, 152,
  155
Obsessive thoughts, 151
Oils and dressings, 208, 222
Optimism, 59–60, 98
Oreo technique, 187–88
Out-of-control feelings, 129, *129*
Overeaters Anonymous, 42
Overeating, 81
Oxytocin, 82, 101

Packaged foods, fast foods, 195–97
Pain relief, 79
Paralysis-analysis, 57–58, 155, 162
Passion, 66, 99
Pasta, 236, 299
Peace, 65, 99, 161–62
Peaceful Protein Pasta, 299
Pep-Me-Up Pizza, 300
Perfectionism, 5, 93, 215
Permanence, 62–63, 132
Personalization, 55–56
Perspective, 56–57
Pervasiveness, 56–57
Pessimism, 58–60
Physical need, of food addiction, 14, 30
Pitfalls, 231. *See also* Mantra pitfalls
 activities, thought patterns, brain
  chemicals and, 47
 anxiety, perfectionism and, 5, 85–86,
  93, 201–2
 attributes for mastering, 63–67
 boosters replacing, 46–48, 53, 81,
  94, 97–98, 117, 182–83, 240
 mantra, weight and, 89, 149–50

Pitfall foods, 5, 16, 47, 49, 52, 231. *See also* Dopamine pitfall foods; Serotonin pitfall foods
  addiction to, 48
  alcohol, 237–38
  caffeine, 114
  diet soda, fruit juice, soda, 239
  disguised, 248–49
  emotional eating of, 154–56
  fat, high levels, saturated, 26, 228
  fruit list of, 237
  manageable, 244–46
  replacing with booster, 97–98, 182–83
  satiety, low, 189, *189*
  self-medication with, 86, 147
  serving sizes, 244–46
  swap list, booster foods for, 246–48
  taste recalibration for replacing, 184
  treats, 229
  weight gain from, 17
  withdrawal of, 48
Pitfall thought patterns, 47, 53–63, 201–2, 215
  actions, feelings and, 88–89, 89, 91, *91*
  changing, 91, 145
  cognitive-behavioral therapy for, 53
  identifying and reframing, 55, 117
  as negative catalyst, 9, 54, *54*
  paralysis-analysis, 57–58, 155, 162
  permanence, 62–63
  personalization, 55–56
  pervasiveness, 56–57
  pessimism, 58–60
  polarization, 60–61
  psychic, 61–62
  Talk to Your Heart technique for, 132–33, 145, 153
Planning meals, 176
Pleasure, 66–67, 163
Polarization, 60–61

Portion sizes, 204–5, 219–20
Positive reinforcement, 100
Power, 65, 126, 161–63
Pride, 65, 99, 148, 161, 163
Productivity, 66, 161
Protein, 206, 218, 220, 298, 299
Prozac, 2
Psychic, 61–62
Psychotherapy, 21
Purpose, 64, 99, 161

Ray, Rachael, 186
Recalibration, of taste, 186–88
  accepting new food for, 98, 188
  bitter, fatty, salty, sweet cravings and, 183–85
  diet soda, to stop habit, 114–15
  Oreo technique, 187–88
  replacing pitfall foods, 184
  supertasters and, 185–86
  taste, temperature, tint, texture, 187
  technique, easy, 186–88
Recipes, 297–303
Relapsing, 241–42
Relationships, weight and, 149
Restrictive diets. *See* Diets, restrictive

Salad dressing, 239
Salmon, 233
Salt
  food tastes stimulated by, 193, 195
  as gateway drug, 194
  habit, breaking of, 195, 197–98
  hypertension from overuse of, 196, 198
  packaged foods, fast foods with, 195–97
  spices, herbs, substitute for, 193, 199–200
  taste recalibration of, 183
Satiety, 188–89
Saturated fat, 26, 228
Schedules, Diet Rehab, 233–34

Index

Seafood, 206, 221

Seductive Soup and Salad, 300

Self-esteem, and serotonin, 20

Self-medication
  binge eating for, 170
  booster food to help with, 86,
    115–16
  dopamine, serotonin and, 115–16,
    216
  with food, 2, 5, 9, 29, 90, 115–16
  with pitfall foods, 86, 115–16, 147
  soda, sugar, caffeine for, 115–16

Serotonin, 20–22
  antidepressants increasing, 2, 11, 79,
    83, 111
  anxiety depleting, 2, 84–85, 85, 101,
    201
  bariatric surgery reducing, 42
  brain chemistry and, 2, 9, 20, 71, 82,
    159–60
  carbohydrates and sugar boost of, 2,
    7, 21, 83, 150, 152, 201–2
  cardiovascular system regulated by,
    78–79
  cigarettes/smoking reducing, 82–83
  cortisol and depletion of, 36–37
  Diet Rehab program, raising, 100,
    201, 202–4, 232
  digestion and, 79
  drugs, boosting levels of, 2–3
  foods, releasing, 147
  hungry for, 71–77
  journals for deficient, 252–55
  mantra "because" challenge list for,
    93–94, 97
  men, higher levels in, 111
  as pain reliever, 79
  restrictive diets depleting, 24–25,
    83
  tolerance, carbohydrates, sugar and,
    79
  withdrawal from sugar, 14, 20, 79
Serotonin, high levels, 71, 98, 100

Serotonin, low levels, 27, 71, 95, 141
  agreeable personalities developed
    from, 84
  anxiety produced by, 2, 78, 84–85,
    101, 201
  anxious thoughts of, 85
  attitudes, behaviors of, 128, 128–29
  binge eating from, 166–67
  boosters for raising, 85, 95–96
  cravings for carbohydrates/sugar in,
    100, 150, 201–2
  depletion of, 24–25
  Diet Rehab program for helping, 232
  emotional eating and, 159–60
  exhaustion from, 115
  food addictions from, 89, 147
  ghrelin, lack of sleep from, 203
  mantra identified for, 87–88, 150
  obsessive behaviors, boosters for,
    143
  obsessive-compulsive disorder from,
    78
  obsessive eating, boosters for, 142,
    145
  overeating, "food coma" from, 81
  pitfall mantras depleting, 87–88, 150
  pitfalls replaced with boosters for, 81
  pitfall thought patterns, creating, 54,
    54, 201–2, 215
  psychotherapy to change, 21
  self-esteem and, 20
  self-medication for, 115–16
  self-starvation and, 149
  sleep problems caused by, 78, 81,
    113, 203
  weight gain from, 81, 89
  women and, 83–84, 111
  worries created by, 201–2
Serotonin booster activities, 6, 79, 96,
    98, 100, 115, 148, 150, 152
  list of, 203–4, 208–13
  mantra booster for, 72, 92, 92, 100,
    208–13

sleep as, 203
soothing activities as, 203–4
spirituality, reconnecting to as, 204
stretching, calming exercises as, 203
Sun, vitamin D as, 203
Serotonin booster foods, 24, 85–86, 97–98, 100, 115, 202–8, 243
Serotonin boosters, 72, 79, 81, 82, 85, 95–96, 150, 152, 204–8
Serotonin norepinephrine reuptake inhibitors (SNRI), 116
Serotonin pitfall foods, 2, 7, 21, 52, 213–14
Serving sizes of pitfall foods, 244–46
Sleep, 20, 78, 81, 113–14, 203
Smoking. See Cigarettes/smoking
Snacks, 243, 302–3
Soda, 239
    diet, 114–15, 116, 239
    self-medication with, 115–16
Soothing activities, 203–4
South Beach Diet, 22, 28, 181
Spices, herbs, 193, 199–200, 208, 223
Spirituality, 204
Splenda, 240
Starch, 203
Starvation mode, 22–23
Strattera, 116
Stress, 2–4, 36–37, 135
Stretching, 203
Sugar, 13
    addiction to, 14, 35
    binge eating and, 166–67
    blood sugar, 80, 100
    cravings, 100, 150, 201–2
    hidden in foods, 100
    insulin resistance and, 80–81
    satiety, low, 188
    self-medication with, 115–16
    serotonin increased by, 2, 7, 21, 152
    tolerance of, 79
    weight gain from, 17
    withdrawal symptoms of, 14, 20, 79
Sun, 203
Supertasters, 185–86
Swap lists, booster foods, 8, 100, 125, 246–48
Sweeteners, 223, 240
Sweet foods, 202–3

Talk to Your Heart technique, 132–33, 145, 153
Tastes, 181–92. See also Recalibration, of taste
Thinness, excessive, 305
Titillating Tacos, 301
Tolerance
    carbohydrate, sugar, 79
    creating addiction, 32–33
    high fat, 19, 19, 22
    weight gain caused by, 33, 81
Treats, 229
Triggers, 155, 169, 173
Tung Fong, 13

Vegan/vegetarian booster foods, finding, 238
Vegetables, 207, 222, 236–37
Vitamin D, 203

Weighing yourself, 177
Weight
    binge eating and, 174
    emotional eating, relationship to, 155
    hypertension and, 196, 198
    mantra and, 87–89, 119–20
    relationships influencing, 149
Weight gain
    compulsive eating and, 13–14
    cortisol and, 36–37
    diet soda causing, 114
    dopamine and, 24–25, 25, 112
    dual deficiencies and, 134

Weight gain (*cont.*)
  food addiction and, 28–30, 120
  genetics and, 38, 94–95
  high-fat, high-sugar pitfall foods and,
    17
  insulin resistance and, 36–37
  restrictive eating and, 22–23, *23*,
    24–25, *25*
  serotonin and, 24–25, *25*, 81, 89
  stress, from, 36–37
  tolerance promoting, 33, 81
  willpower and, 14, 22, 25
  women and, 112
  yo-yo dieting and, 29, 37
Weight loss
  bariatric surgery for, 25–26, 41–42
  and eating normally, 170
  emotional eating, 154–57
  and mantras, 149–50
  sleep booster, 203
  sustainable, 25, 93
Wellbutrin, 3, 113, 116
"What's right" glasses, 94
Whole grains, seeds, 205, 220
Willpower
  food addiction and, 7, 14, 16, 30

restrictive diets and, 22
weight gain and, 14, 22, 25
Withdrawal
  Diet Rehab program, 46, 48
  dopamine, symptoms of, 2, 17–18
  dual deficiencies and, 129–30
  foods, activities, thought patterns
    and, 46
  gradual detox and, 45–46
  symptoms of, 14, 20, 34–35, 79
Women
  antidepressants, serotonin-targeted
    for, 11
  depression risk of, 83, 111
  dopamine, low levels and weight
    gain in, 112
  restrictive diets and, 83–84
  serotonin, low levels in, 83–84, 111

Xylitol, 240

Yo-yo dieting, 29, 37, 178

Zoloft, 2
the Zone, 28
Zyban, 25